AF573844

Atlas of Foot and Ankle Sonography

Atlas of Foot and Ankle Sonography

Ronald Adler, PhD, MD
Attending Radiologist
Chief, Division of Ultrasound and Body Imaging
Hospital for Special Surgery
Professor of Radiology
Weill Medical College of Cornell University
New York, NY

Carolyn M. Sofka, MD
Assistant Attending Radiologist
Department of Radiology and Body Imaging
Hospital for Special Surgery
Assistant Professor of Radiology
Weill Medical College of Cornell University
New York, NY

Rock G. Positano, DPM, MSc, MPH
Director
Non-Operative Foot and Ankle Center
Hospital for Special Surgery
Co-Director
The Foot Center
Orthopedic Trauma Service
New York Presbyterian Hospital
Weill Cornell Medical Center
Hospital for Special Surgery
Clinical Assistant Professor
Department of Surgery
Weill Medical College of Cornell University
New York, NY

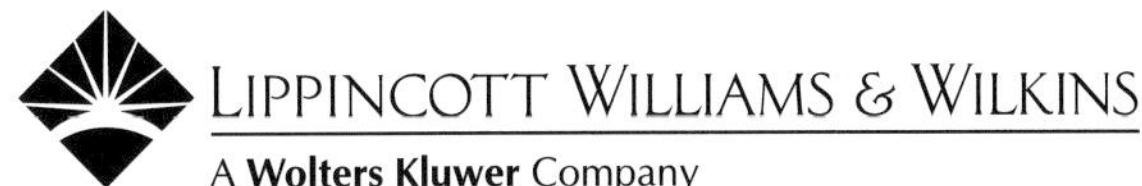
LIPPINCOTT WILLIAMS & WILKINS
A Wolters Kluwer Company
Philadelphia • Baltimore • New York • London
Buenos Aires • Hong Kong • Sydney • Tokyo

Acquisitions Editor: Lisa McAllister
Developmental Editor: Joanne Bersin
Supervising Editor: Mary Ann McLaughlin
Production Editor: Richard Rothschild, Print Matters, Inc.
Manufacturing Manager: Colin J. Warnock
Cover Designer: Christine Jenny
Compositor: Compset, Inc.
Printer: Maple Press

530 Walnut Street
Philadelphia, PA 19106 USA
LWW.com

Printed in the USA

Library of Congress Cataloging-in-Publication Data
Adler, Ronald.
Atlas of foot and ankle sonography / Ronald Adler, Carolyn M. Sofka, Rock G. Positano.
p. ; cm.
Includes bibliographical references and index.
ISBN 0-7817-4769-4 (alk. paper)
1. Foot—Ultrasonic imaging—Atlases. 2. Ankle—Ultrasonic imaging—Atlases. I. Sofka, Carolyn M. II. Positano, Rock G. III. Title.
[DNLM: 1. Ankle—ultrasonography—Atlases. 2. Foot—ultrasonography—Atlases. 3. Foot Diseases—ultrasonography—Atlases. WE 17 A237a 2004]
RC951.A34 2004
617.5'85'07544—dc22

2004040948

---

10 9 8 7 6 5 4 3 2 1

Contents

Preface

Advances in ultrasound technology have resulted in an expanded role of ultrasound in the evaluation of foot and ankle disorders. High-resolution imaging afforded by the current generation of ultrasound scanners produces exquisite images of tendons, muscles, nerves, and ligaments in real-time. As a result, these structures may be assessed dynamically while being imaged, a feature that is unique to ultrasound. Likewise, the real-time nature of ultrasound allows direct visualization of needle placement during the performance of therapeutic interventions. The presence of indwelling hardware does not interfere with the functional and anatomic evaluation of the foot and ankle. These improvements along with economic factors and availability make ultrasound an ideal diagnostic tool. As such, the efficacy of ultrasound has been compared to other modalities, in particular magnetic resonance imaging, as a cost-efficient imaging alternative.

In what follows, ultrasound imaging of the foot and ankle is illustrated, beginning with discussions of technique and the technical factors that the imager should be aware of. Some general principles of musculoskeletal ultrasound are then discussed. The foot and ankle subject is arbitrarily divided into four anatomic regions: forefoot, midfoot, ankle and hindfoot. Additional sections dealing with miscellaneous abnormalities, i.e., masses, foreign bodies, etc., and a specific interventional section are included to complete the book. We hope that this serves as an atlas, displaying both normal ultrasound anatomy as well as a variety of common (and some uncommon) pathologic states. Material has been presented in such a way as to be amenable to both imagers and referring clinicians alike. We have concentrated mainly on gray scale imaging with extensive use of extended field of view imaging, which is a relatively new development in ultrasound. The latter permits better depiction of anatomic relationships as well as the extent of a lesion. We have also emphasized the interventional aspects of ultrasound, which serves as an important advantage of its use of ultrasound.

Acknowledgments

Special thanks to April Roland, who was instrumental in helping to put the manuscript together.

—Ron Adler

I would like to thank Riana F. Positano for her support in my work.

—Rock Positano

I thank all of my colleagues and staff in the Department of Radiology, particularly Helene Pavlov, MD, FACR, and Ron Adler, PhD, MD, for their support. As teachers, examples and friends, they have been an invaluable resource. I also thank my family for their love and generosity of spirit—their patience, counsel and strength have been an inspiration.

—Carolyn Sofka

1

General Principles

SONOGRAPHIC APPEARANCES

Diagnostic sonography of the foot and ankle requires appropriate imaging equipment as well as patient positioning. In general, a medium- to high-frequency linear transducer (7.5 to 15 MHz) can be used to evaluate most structures about the foot and ankle.

Tendons are normally seen as multiple hyperechoic (bright) interfaces arranged in a parallel linear fashion, invested within a synovial lined sheath or by dense connective tissue (paratenon) (1,2) (Fig. 1-1). Because of this highly ordered fibrillar arrangement of extracellular collagen giving rise to these multiple interfaces, tendons display an acoustic property known as *anisotropy* (3) (Fig. 1-2). In practice, this means that slight angulation or obliquity of an ultrasound transducer can result in a hypoechoic appearance of the tendon being examined, leading the sonographer to believe there is tendinosis or even a tear of the tendon (4).

Tendinopathy or tendinosis is demonstrated with sonography as decreased echogenicity of the tendon, often with tendon enlargement (1) (Fig. 1-3). Hypoechoic intratendinous clefts may also be seen. Measurements of various tendons have been suggested as pathologic, but it must be remembered that gender, size and training can contribute to tendon thickness. The tendon may lose its normal sharp outline, displaying indistinct margins. Focal tendinosis displays localized areas of thickening and hypoechogenicity. It has been shown that internal changes in tendon morphology can often be diagnosed earlier with high-resolution sonography than with magnetic resonance imaging, in the absence of tailored protocols and surface coils (5,6). High-frequency transducers, which vary between 10 and 15 MHz, can have an in-plane resolution of 200 to 450 μm (5).

Tenosynovitis is seen as a pathologic quantity of fluid or thickening of the tendon sheath (1) (Fig. 1-4). This may be secondary to inflammation, infection, acute trauma, or an effusion within an adjacent joint. Increased peritendinous vascularity is frequently evident on power Doppler imaging and may be striking relative to the amount of fluid or synovial thickening (7).

Complete tendon rupture is easily recognized in the acute phase both clinically and sonographically (Fig. 1-5). The tendon retracts, and the gap between the retracted ends may be filled with hematoma. The tendon itself may appear diffusely thickened, heterogeneous, and nodular in contour. Partial rupture is similar in that there is discontinuity in the parallel linear echoes of the tendon, with the gap filled by material of variable, but usually decreased, echogenicity (Fig. 1-6). Because there are some remaining intact fibrils, there may be only minimal retraction in a partial tear. This manifests as a contour deformity or focal thinning. Partial tears may also manifest as splits paralleling the long axis of a tendon (Figs. 1-7 and 1-8). This is particularly prevalent in the ankle.

(Text continues on page 5)

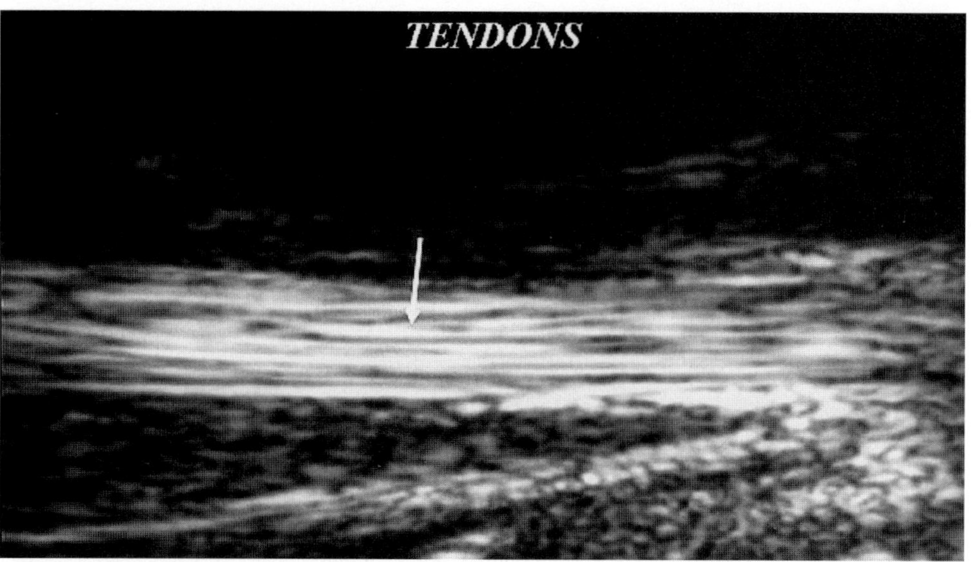

FIG. 1-1. Sonographic appearance of a normal tendon. The tendon appears hyperechoic with a fine internal linear fibrillar architecture (*arrow*).

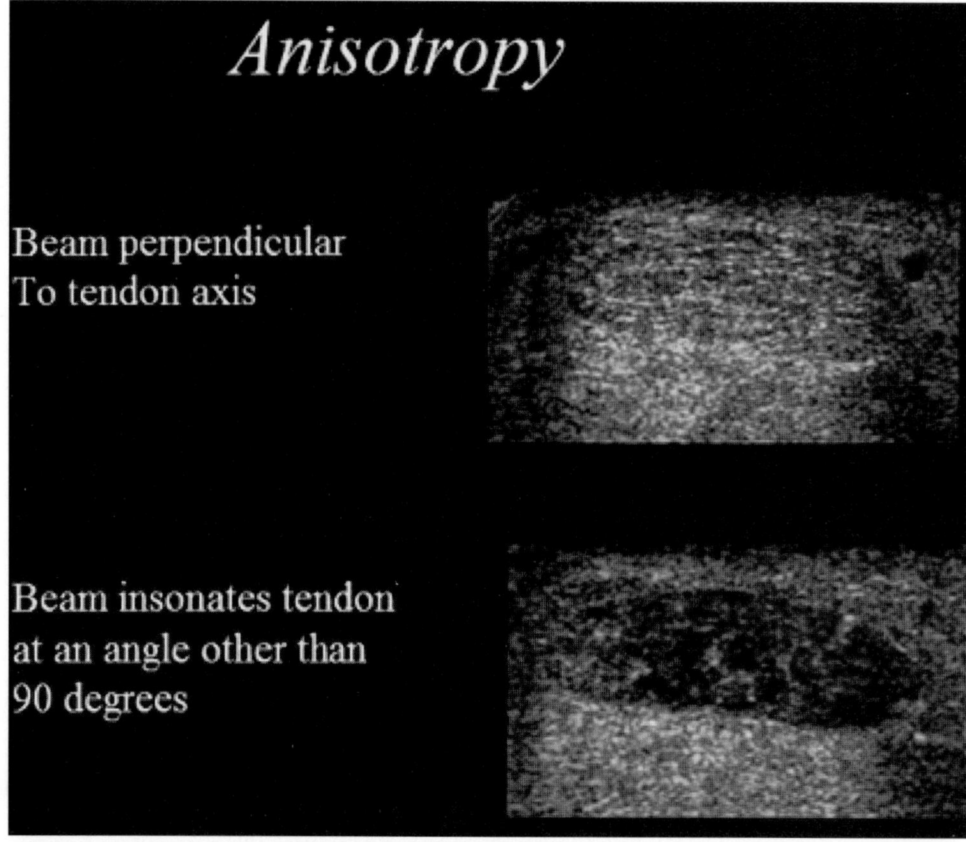

FIG. 1-2. Tendons are inherently anisotropic tissues. When the ultrasound beam is held directly perpendicular to a normal tendon as seen in cross section, the tendon should be fairly homogeneously hyperechoic (**top**). If the ultrasound beam is angled even slightly away from the perpendicular, the tendon will appear progressively more hypoechogenic (**bottom**). Proper technique is important to avoid a false diagnosis of tendinosis.

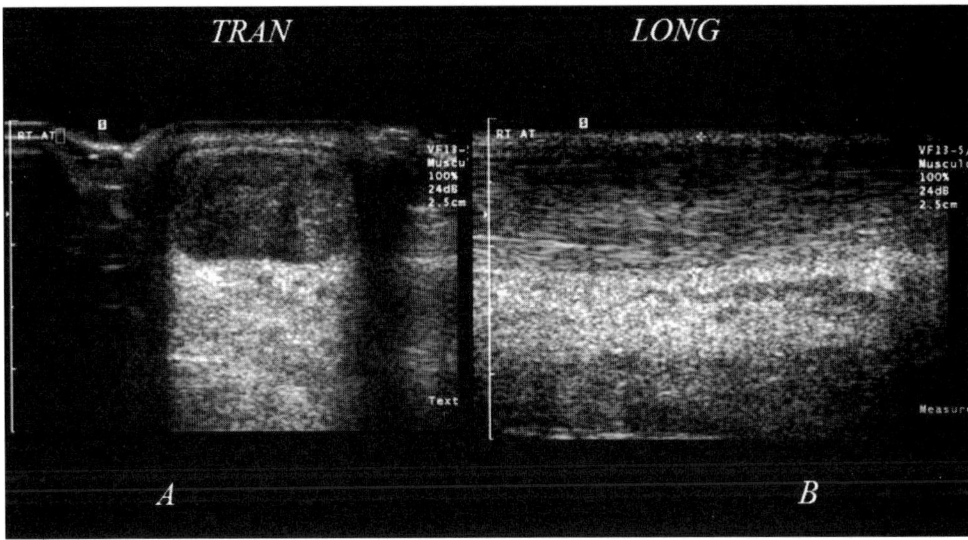

FIG. 1-3. Transverse (**A**) and longitudinal (**B**) ultrasound images displaying an enlarged inhomogeneous Achilles tendon, typically seen in tendinosis. Note that the underlying fibrillar architecture is preserved.

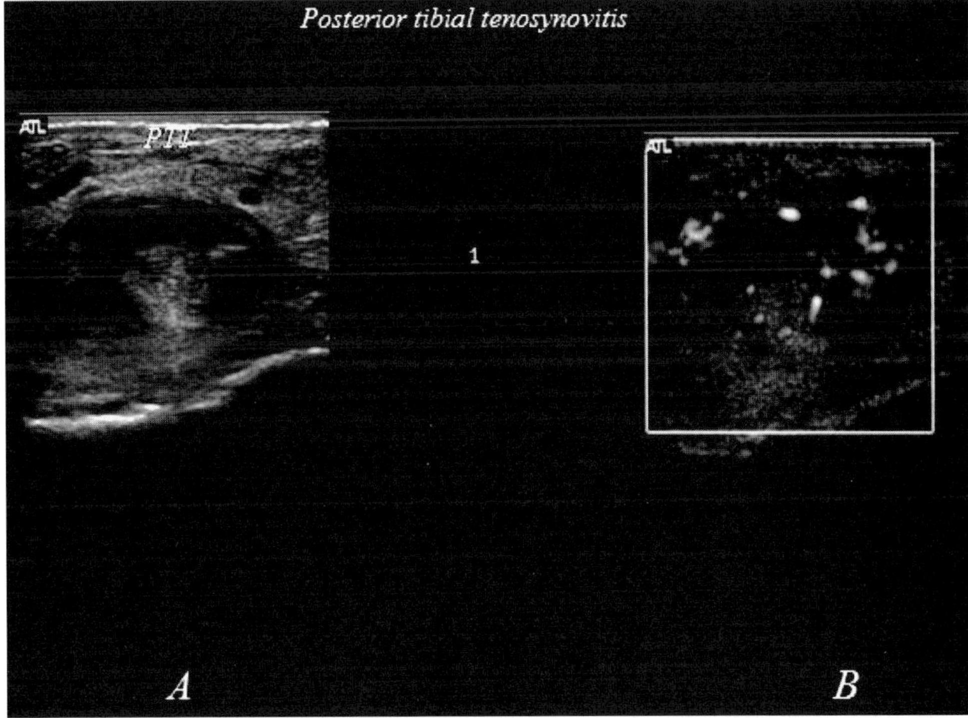

FIG. 1-4. In tenosynovitis, there is distention of the tendon sheath by either fluid or thickened synovium (**A**). The tendon may be abnormal, as in this case, but need not be. The distinction between fluid and synovial thickening may be difficult. Use of power Doppler to display the inherent vascularity of inflamed synovium (**B**) may be of value in distinguishing these entities.

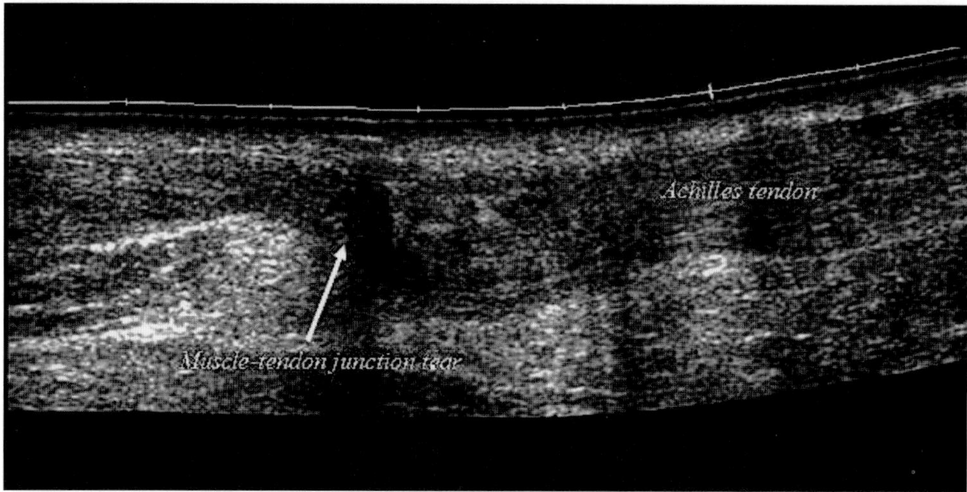

FIG. 1-5. Full-thickness tears are characterized by a hypoechoic defect traversing the entire width of the tendon (*arrow*). There can be variable degrees of retraction of the tendon ends with "balling up" and displacement. This case displays a complete tear of the Achilles tendon at the myotendinous junction. The distal tendon stump (**right** of the *arrow*) is thickened and displaced inferiorly. The proximal stump (**left**) is thinned. The echogenic material filling the gap likely corresponds to herniated fat.

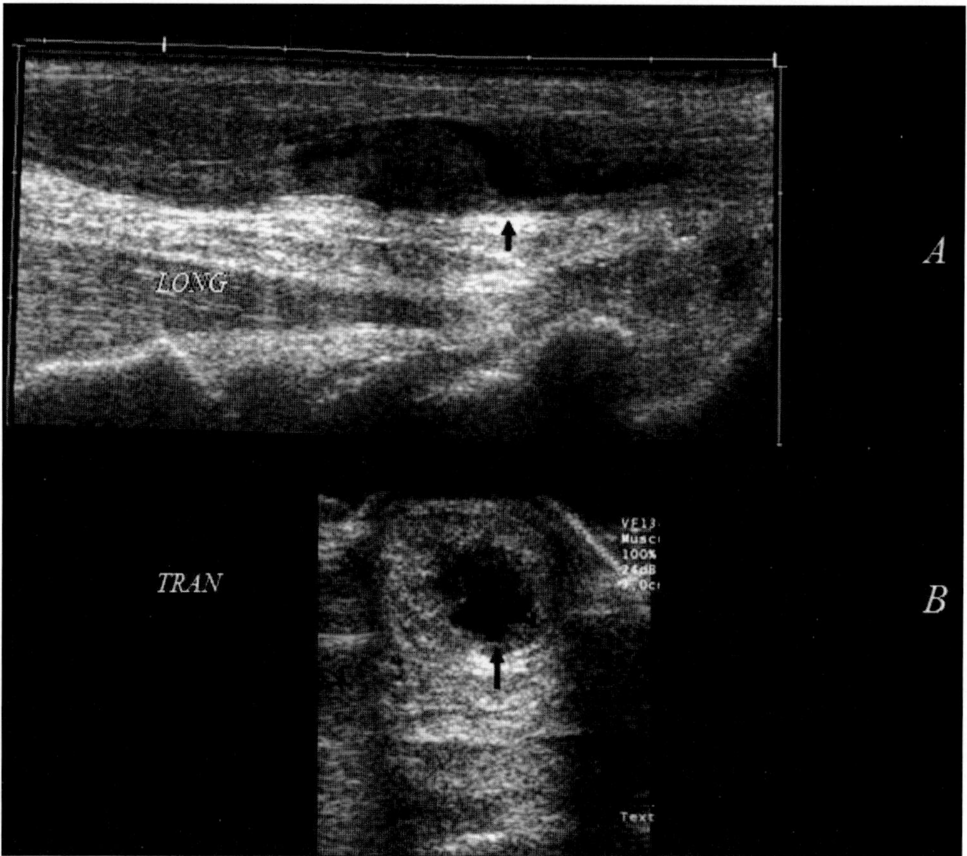

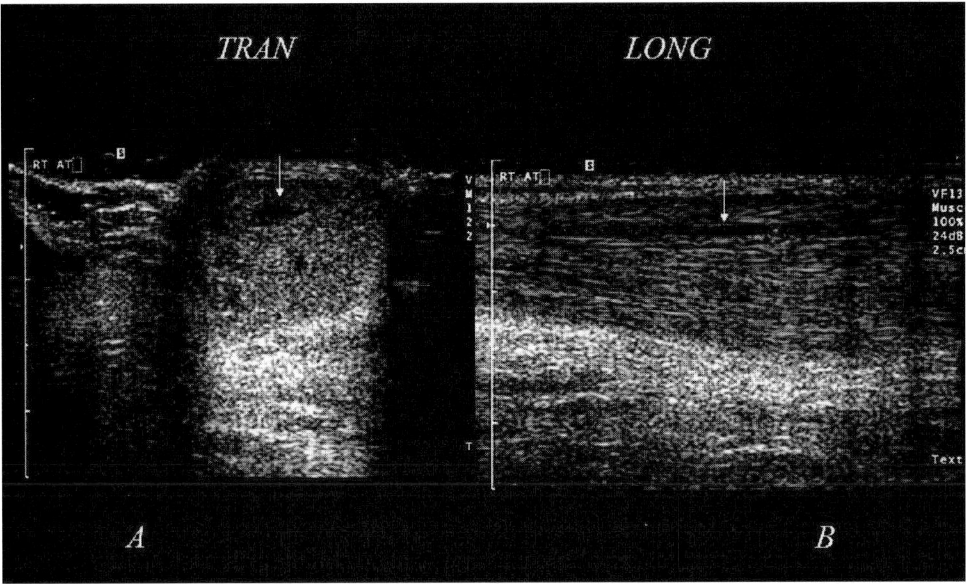

FIG. 1-7. Tears may be entirely intrasubstance, as in this case. The Achilles tendon is displayed in transverse (**A**) and longitudinal (**B**) planes. The tendon is enlarged and inhomogeneous, containing a longitudinal-oriented, intrasubstance tear (split) denoted by the *arrow*.

Peripheral nerves, such as the posterior tibial nerve, can be visualized with sonography using high-frequency transducers. Peripheral nerves are hypoechoic linear bands of tissue encased by thin echogenic fibroadipose layers (epineurium) with speckled curvilinear hyperechoic foci (endoneurium) surrounding the hypoechoic nerve fascicles (8) (Fig. 1-9). Ligaments are seen as tightly compact echogenic bands of tissue (Fig. 1-10).

Other structures within the foot and ankle that can be evaluated with sonography include cortical bone (Fig. 1-11), which is seen as a highly reflective echogenic linear structure demonstrating posterior acoustic shadowing, and articular cartilage, which is uniformly thick and hypoechoic in the normal state (9). Muscle appears hypoechoic with fine linear internal echogenic structures, corresponding to fibroadipose connective tissue separating muscle fascicles (perimysium).

(Text continues on page 9)

FIG. 1-6. Partial-thickness tears arise from either superficial or deep margins of the tendon, or they may be entirely intrasubstance. Tears often occur in the setting of preexisting tendinosis. The current case illustrates longitudinal (**A**) and transverse (**B**) views of the Achilles tendon. The tendon is enlarged and inhomogeneous, with a discretely marginated hypoechoic defect (*arrow*) arising from the deep margin, corresponding to a partial tear. The tear does not extend to the superficial margin of the tendon.

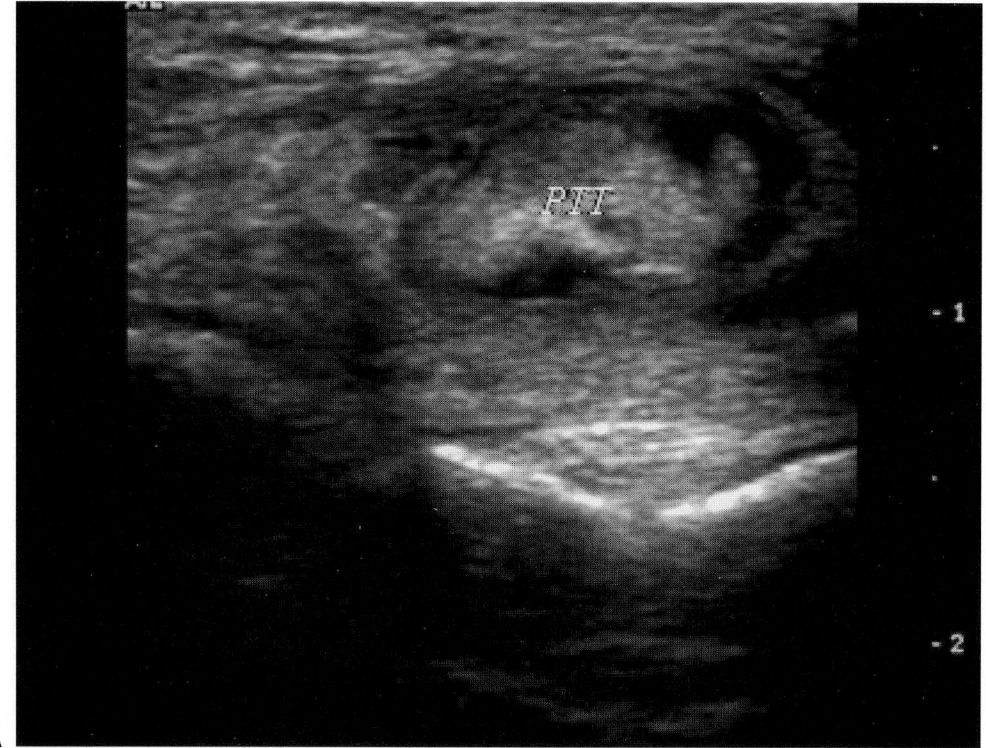

A

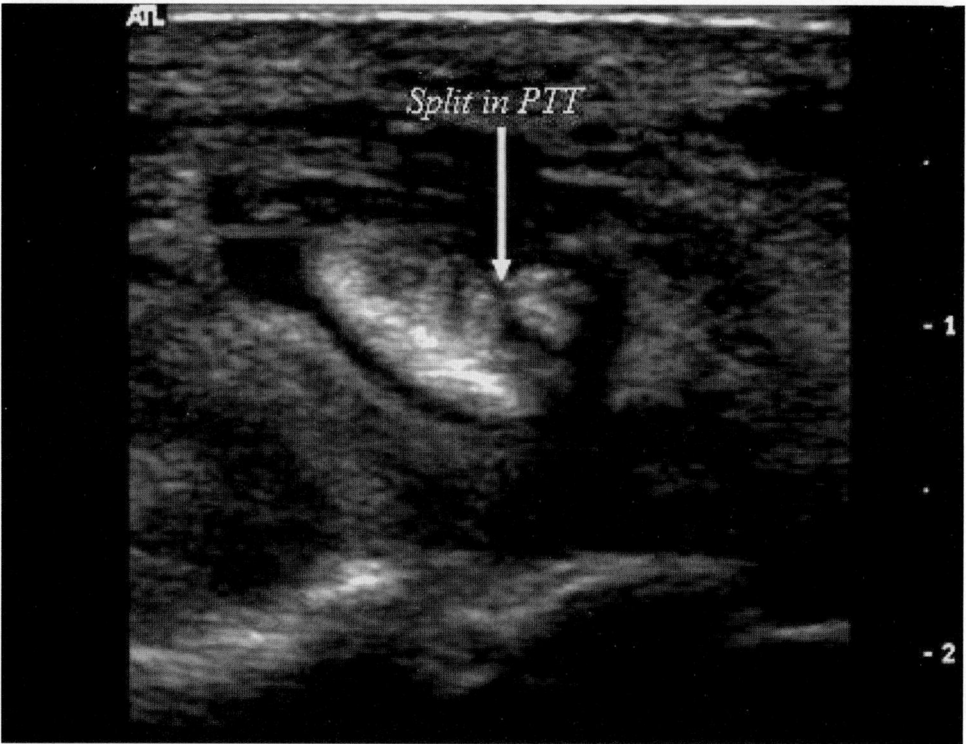

B

FIG. 1-8. Splits are best seen in short axis as illustrated in this case. **A, B:** Short axis views of the posterior tibial tendon in different patients with medial ankle pain. In each case, the tendon is inhomogeneous with a surrounding tendon sheath effusion. **A:** A discrete V-shaped split is present along the superficial margin of the tendon. **B:** Multiple splits are evident along the superficial margin of the tendon, one extending to the other side of the tendon (*arrow*).

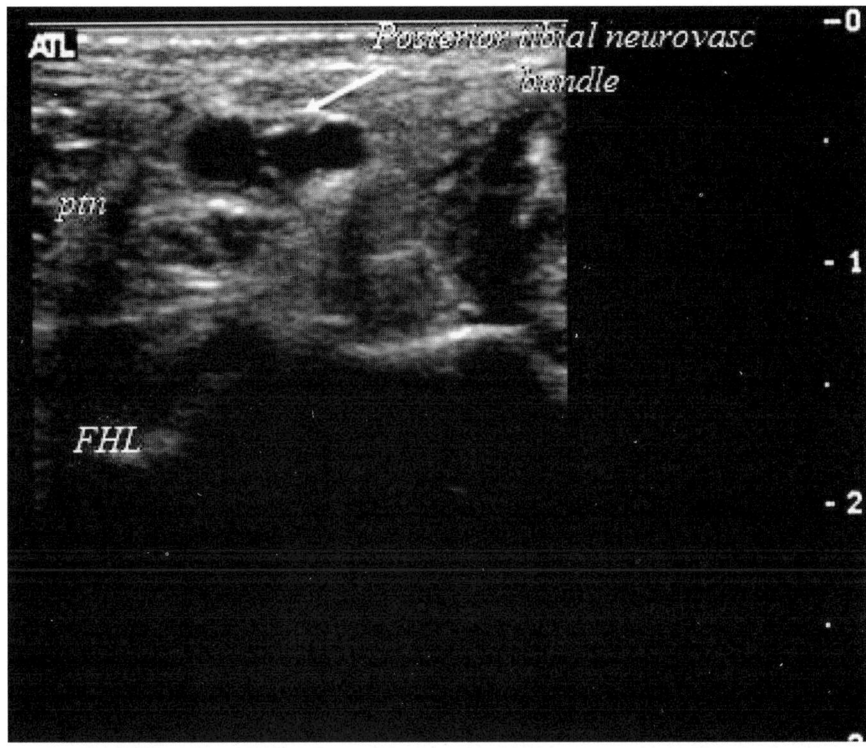

FIG. 1-9. Transverse image over the medial compartment of the ankle shows the neurovascular structures here. The three rounded anechoic structures correspond to a central posterior tibial artery and adjacent veins. Below these vessels, there is an elliptical hypoechoic structure corresponding to the posterior tibial nerve (PTN). The nerve displays an echogenic periphery, corresponding to the epineurium. The flexor hallucis longus tendon (FHL) is seen in short axis.

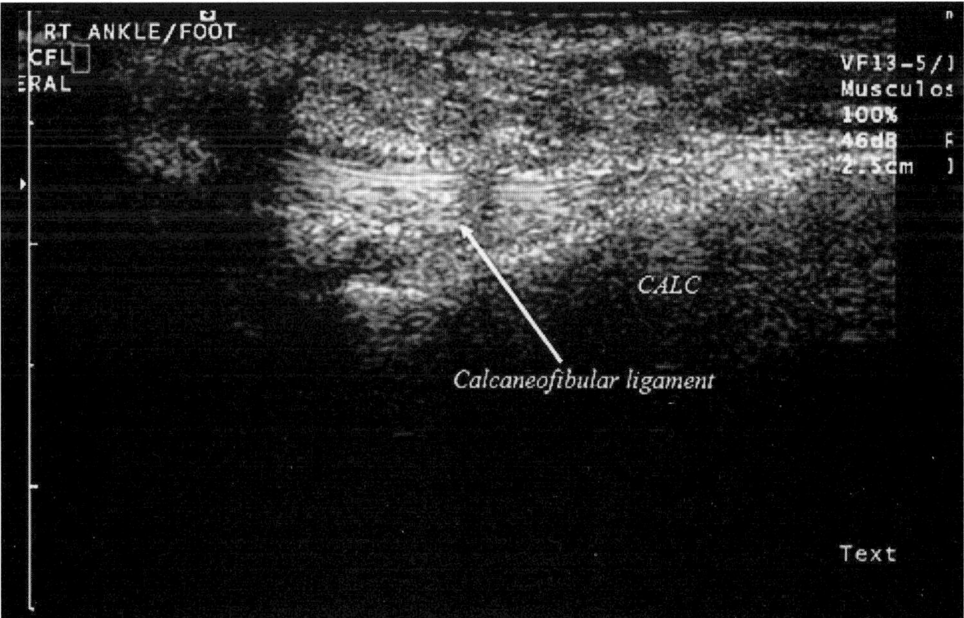

FIG. 1-10. Ligaments are characteristically echogenic and may demonstrate a fibrillar architecture similar to tendons. In this case, the normal calcaneofibular ligament is shown (*arrow*), which displays these properties. The calcaneus (calc) is labeled.

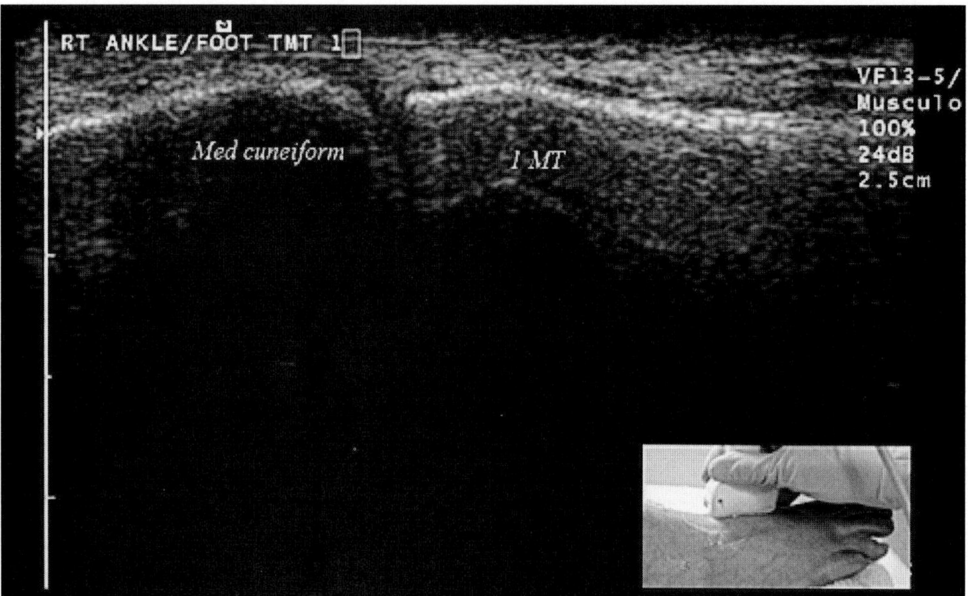

A

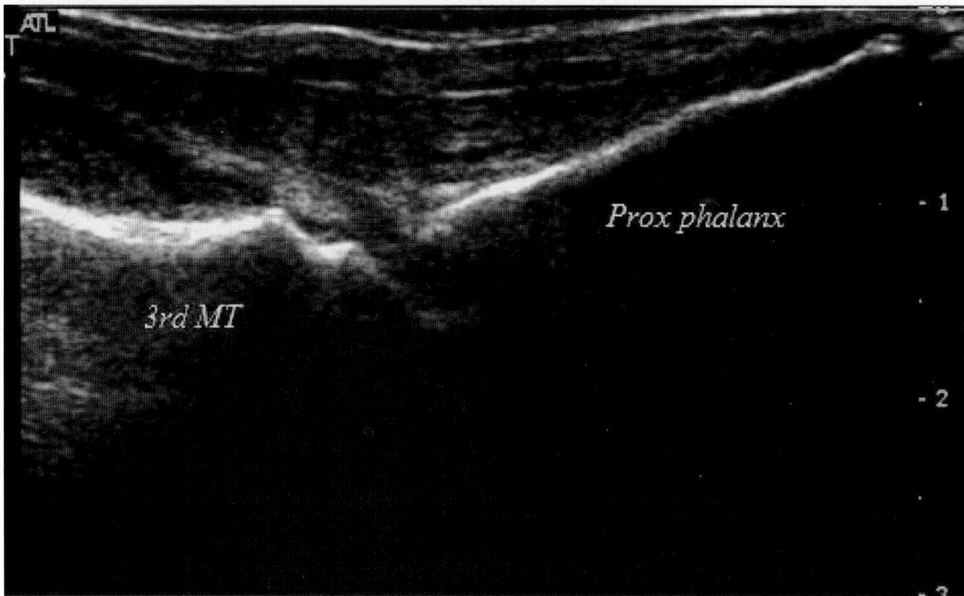

B

FIG. 1-11. Bones are echogenic surfaces that display posterior acoustic shadowing. This results from the absence of significant sound transmission beyond the cortical margin. **A:** The transducer is placed along the first tarsometatarsal joint (**bottom right**). The medial cuneiform and first metatarsal are labeled. Both bones display strong specular (reflective) surfaces with an apparent discontinuity at the joint line. **B:** The margins of the third metatarsal phalangeal joint (labeled) are displayed. Again, no soft tissue detail is evident below the cortical specular echoes owing to lack of sound penetration.

TECHNICAL CONSIDERATIONS

Recent technical advances have greatly improved diagnostic accuracy in the sonographic evaluation of the musculoskeletal system. Tissue harmonic imaging derives from the nonlinear dependence of the speed of sound in soft tissues. The second harmonic component of the transmitted frequency is detected by the ultrasound transducer. The resulting tissue harmonic images display noise reduction and less near-field artifact (10). Axial resolution is improved, resulting in a crisper image, with better definition of internal architecture and tissue interfaces. Compound imaging also can achieve improvements in tissue boundary detection, by averaging the returning ultrasound beam from several different look-angles. This also works to decrease speckle, which refers to the inherent "graininess" encountered with conventional sonography (11,12).

Extended field of view imaging produces a panoramic image of an anatomic region using a single sweep of the transducer (13,14). This allows an image to be produced that displays anatomic information well beyond a conventional two-dimensional gray scale image, without significant loss of image resolution (Fig. 1-12). Extended field of view imaging can more than double the size of the image, displaying as much as 60 cm on a single image (13).

Power Doppler imaging can provide important information with regard to areas of active inflammation (Fig. 1-4). The higher sensitivity of power Doppler compared with conventional color Doppler makes it more useful in evaluating areas of inflammation in the musculoskeletal system (15,16). It has particular advantages in distinguishing bland tendon sheath effusions from inflamed synovium (7). Metallic implants, screws, and needles present a characteristic appearance on ultrasound, demonstrating strongly reflective specular surfaces with a posterior ring-down artifact (Fig. 1-13). Moreover, the presence of metal does not adversely affect assessment of the overlying soft tissues.

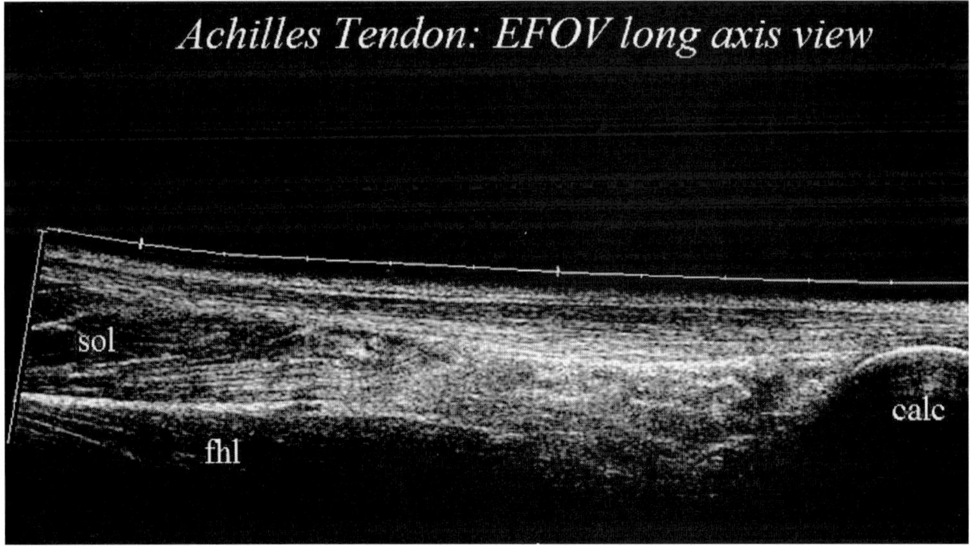

FIG. 1-12. Extended field-of-view imaging allows for a global overview of an anatomic region with a continuous in-plane sweep of the ultrasound transducer. The Achilles tendon, for example, can be imaged and displayed from the muscle–tendon junction [the soleus muscle (sol) is indicated] to the calcaneal insertion (calc). The flexor hallucis longus muscle belly (fhl) is also indicated for reference.

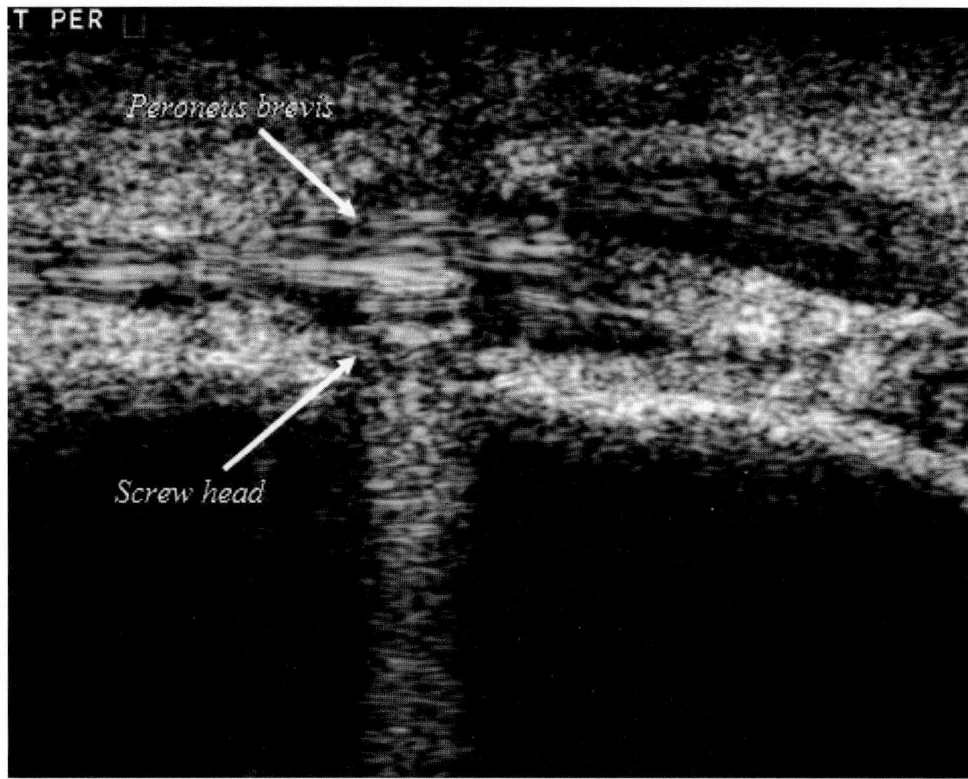

A

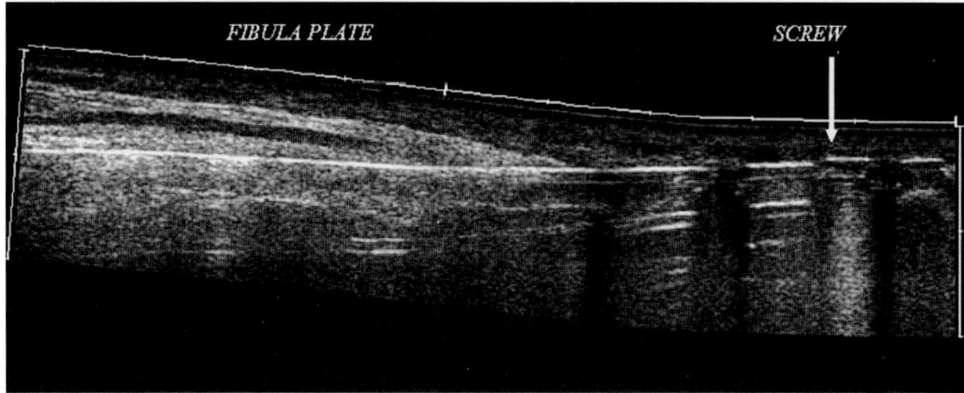

B

FIG. 1-13. Metal displays a characteristic appearance on ultrasound, echogenic with a strong posterior ring-down artifact (sometimes referred to as a "dirty shadow"). **A:** Longitudinal ultrasound image along the lateral joint line in a patient who is status post internal fixation of a calcaneal fracture with focal lateral ankle pain. This longitudinal image demonstrates impingement of the peroneus brevis by one of the screw heads in the calcaneus (labeled). **B:** This patient has an indwelling fibular plate, displayed in this extended field-of-view image. Rather than the typical shadow produced by cortical bone, an extensive ring-down artifact is present, helping to identify this as a metallic object. An empty screw hole is evident as a discontinuity in the plate. A screw in a distal hole is indicated (*arrow*).

REFERENCES

1. Martinoli C, Bianchi S, Derchi LE. Tendon and nerve sonography. *Radiol Clin North Am* 1999;37:691–711.
2. Martinoli C, Derchi LE, Pastorino C, et al. Analysis of echotexture of tendons with ultrasound. *Radiology* 1993;186:839–843.
3. Jacobson JA, van Holsbeeck MT. Musculoskeletal ultrasound. *Orthop Clin North Am* 1998;29:135–165.
4. Crass JR, van de Vegte GL, Harkavy LA. Tendon echogenicity: ex vivo study. *Radiology* 1998;167:499–501.
5. Erickson SJ. High-resolution imaging of the musculoskeletal system. *Radiology* 1997;205:593–618.
6. Jacobson JA. Ultrasound in sports medicine. *Radiol Clin North Am* 2002;40(2):363–386.
7. Newman JS, Adler RS, Bude RO, et al. Detection of soft tissue hyperemia: value of power Doppler sonography. *AJR Am J Roentgenol* 1994;163:385–389.
8. Thain LMF, Downey DB. Sonography of peripheral nerves: technique, anatomy, and pathology. *Ultrasound Q* 2002;18(4):225–245.
9. Adler RS. Bone and articular cartilage. *Clin Diagn Ultrasound* 1995; 30:59–72.
10. Rosenthal SJ, Jones PH, Wetzel LH. Phase inversion tissue harmonic sonographic imaging: a clinical utility study. *AJR Am J Roentgenol* 2001;176:1393–1398.
11. Entrekin RR, Porter BA, Sillesen HH, et al. Real-time spatial compound imaging: application to breast, vascular, and musculoskeletal ultrasound. *Semin Ultrasound CT MRI* 2001;22(1):50–64.
12. Lin DC, Nazarian LN, O'Kane, PL, et al. Advantages of real-time spatial compound sonography of the musculoskeletal system versus conventional sonography. *AJR Am J Roentgenol* 2002;179:1629–1631.
13. Barbarie JE, Wong AD, Cooperberg PL, et al. Extended field-of-view sonography in musculoskeletal disorders. *AJR Am J Roentgenol* 1998;171:751–757.
14. Lin EC, Middleton WD, Teefey SA. Extended field of view sonography in musculoskeletal imaging. *J Ultrasound Med* 1999;18:147–152.
15. Newman JS, Adler RS. Power Doppler sonography: applications in musculoskeletal imaging. *Semin Musculoskel Radiol* 1998;2(3):331–339.
16. Martinoli C, Pretolesi F, Crespi G, et al. Power Doppler sonography: clinical applications. *Eur J Radiol* 1998;28:S133–S140.

2

Forefoot

CLINICAL CONSIDERATIONS

Ultrasound is capable of providing the physician with diagnostic information. All too often, the clinician has been treating the "wrong" condition, only to find, for example, that the capsulitis being treated is in fact a neuroma or a Freiberg's infraction of the second metatarsal. Magnetic resonance imaging (MRI) examination of the forefoot in these cases can be negative for the presence of neuroma if specialized surface coils are not used. The most common indication for sonographic evaluation of the forefoot is for metatarsalgia and neuroma. Causes of metatarsalgia that can be evaluated with sonography include Morton's neuroma, intermetatarsal bursae, stress fractures, and joint-related synovitis (1).

The presence of foreign bodies, adventitial bursae, and masses are readily evaluated with sonography. Fluoroscopy and conventional radiographs have been traditionally used to diagnose standard foreign bodies. However, not all foreign bodies are radiopaque. For example, glass and wood fragments generally are not revealed on x-ray or fluoroscopy, but diagnostic ultrasound is able to clearly make the determination of their presence. The clinician can use this information to locate the foreign body or debris from a wound effectively.

A common error in clinical practice is injection of the wrong web space when a neuroma is suspected clinically. Patients present with a history of undergoing "blind" injections into the second web space when the neuroma is in the third web space. Also, it is not uncommon to have concomitant neuromas in both the second and third web spaces. Patients often present after removal of a neuroma from the second web space, only to be told that a neuroma was also in the third web space. Diagnostic ultrasound imaging reduces the occurrence of this common error.

The imaging evaluation of pregnant women also poses a clinical challenge in the presence of injury. Ultrasound is safe to both the fetus and mother, and fractures and soft tissue injuries are easily and safely diagnosed and then treated.

ULTRASOUND EVALUATION

General evaluation of the forefoot is typically performed using a medium-frequency (7.5 MHz) linear transducer. A higher-frequency (10 to 15 MHz) transducer can be employed for more detailed evaluation of superficial tendons (e.g., extensor digitorum longus and extensor hallucis longus), to evaluate for possible retained foreign body, and to evaluate the margins of the metatarsophalangeal and interphalangeal joints.

For diagnosis of Morton's neuroma, evaluation of the intermetatarsal web spaces should be performed from both the plantar and dorsal aspects of the forefoot (Fig. 2-1). A transaxial view at the same level demonstrates the echogenic metatarsal bones in short

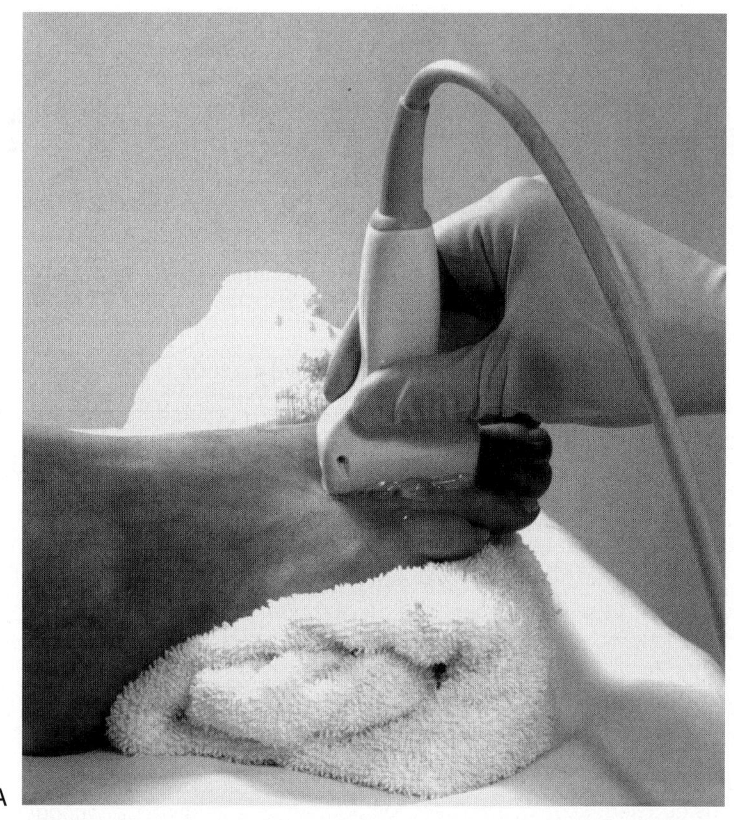

A

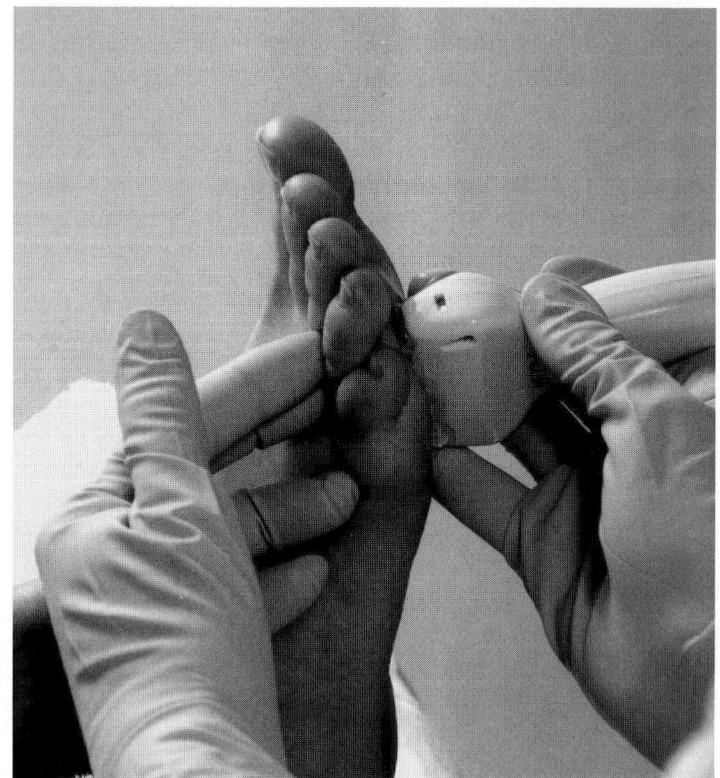

B

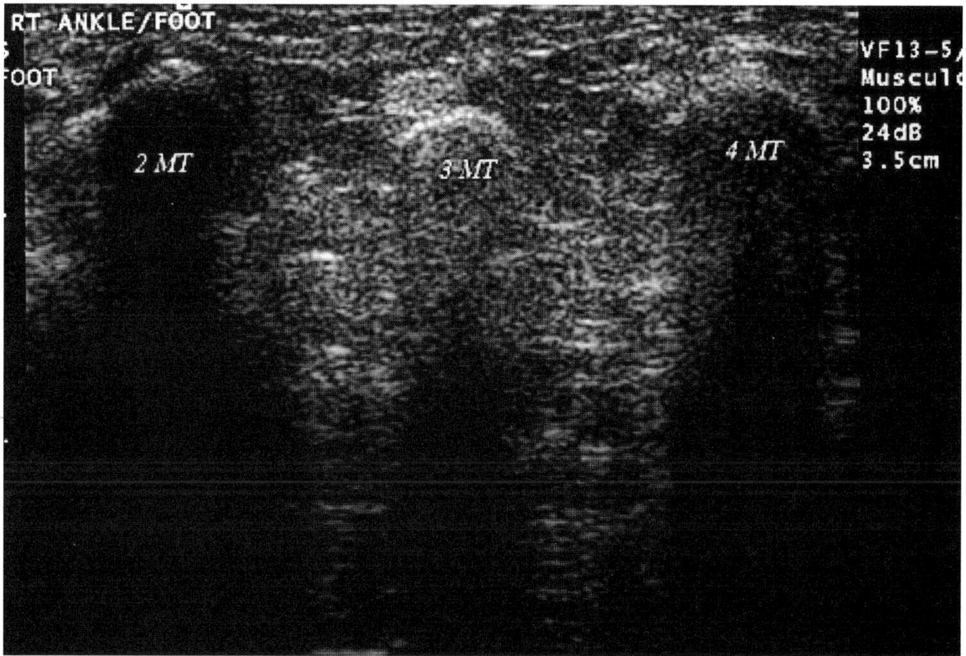

FIG. 2-2. Normal transverse appearance of the forefoot, at the level of the metatarsal heads. The metatarsals (labeled) seen in cross section demonstrate a curvilinear echogenic interface with posterior acoustic shadowing. The intermetatarsal web spaces are normally uniformly hyperechoic because they normally contain only fat, interdigital nerves, and small vessels.

axis with posterior acoustic shadowing; interposed within the hyperechoic intermetatarsal web space, fat should be normally visualized (Fig. 2-2). A longitudinal view of the intermetatarsal web space should normally demonstrate fairly homogeneous echogenic fat only (Fig. 2-3). Morton's neuromas are seen at sonography as discrete round hypoechoic masses in the web spaces replacing the normally hyperechoic interdigital fat (2–4) (Figs. 2-4 to 2-6). In our experience, these occur mostly in the second and third web spaces, occasionally in the first web space, and rarely in the forth web space. A tubular hypoechoic structure can be seen associated with the neuroma, consistent with an enlarged interdigital nerve (Fig. 2-6). Also, adventitial bursae can be seen in association with Morton's neuromas (5) or as an isolated finding (Figs. 2-6 to 2–8). Applying pressure to the margin of the web space opposite the transducer while imaging the web space can help distinguish bursae from the adjacent neuromas because the bursae compress with pressure, but the neuromas do not. Recurrent, or stump, neuromas can also be identified with ultrasound (6). Occasionally, other masses may mimic neuromas or produce similar symptoms,

FIG. 2-1. A: Technique for obtaining longitudinal images of the intermetatarsal web space, using a dorsal approach. The web spaces should be imaged transversely as well as longitudinally, approximately at the level of the metatarsal heads. **B:** Scanning along the plantar aspect of the web space while applying pressure on the dorsal aspect can help distinguish a noncompressible neuroma from a compressible intermetatarsal bursa.

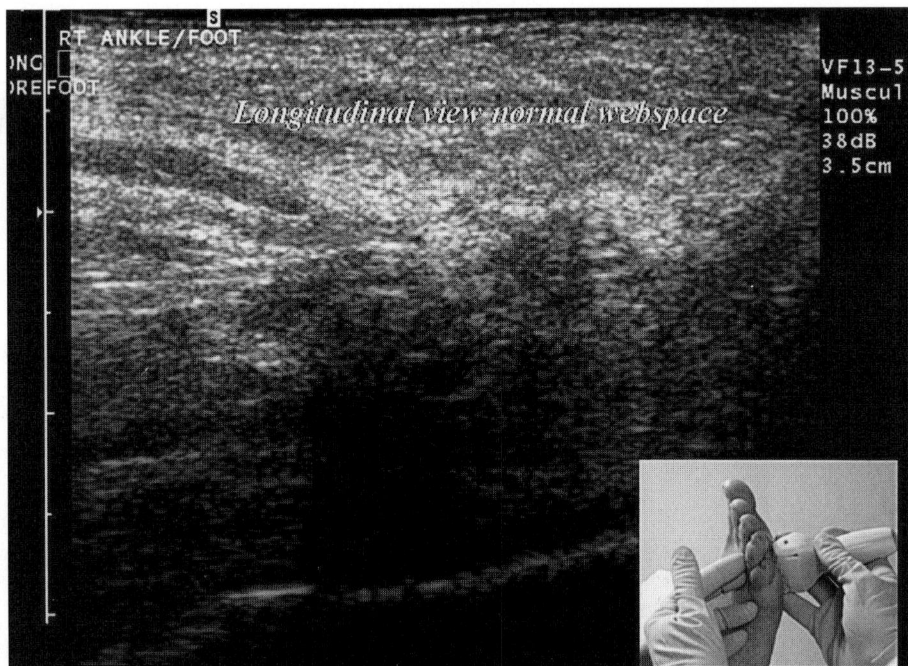

FIG. 2-3. Normally, the intermetatarsal web spaces should contain only hyperechoic fat, as depicted here. Dorsal compression can be helpful to assess the margins of a neuroma. It is when this normally hyperechoic fat is replaced with an incompressible hypoechoic mass that a neuroma can be diagnosed.

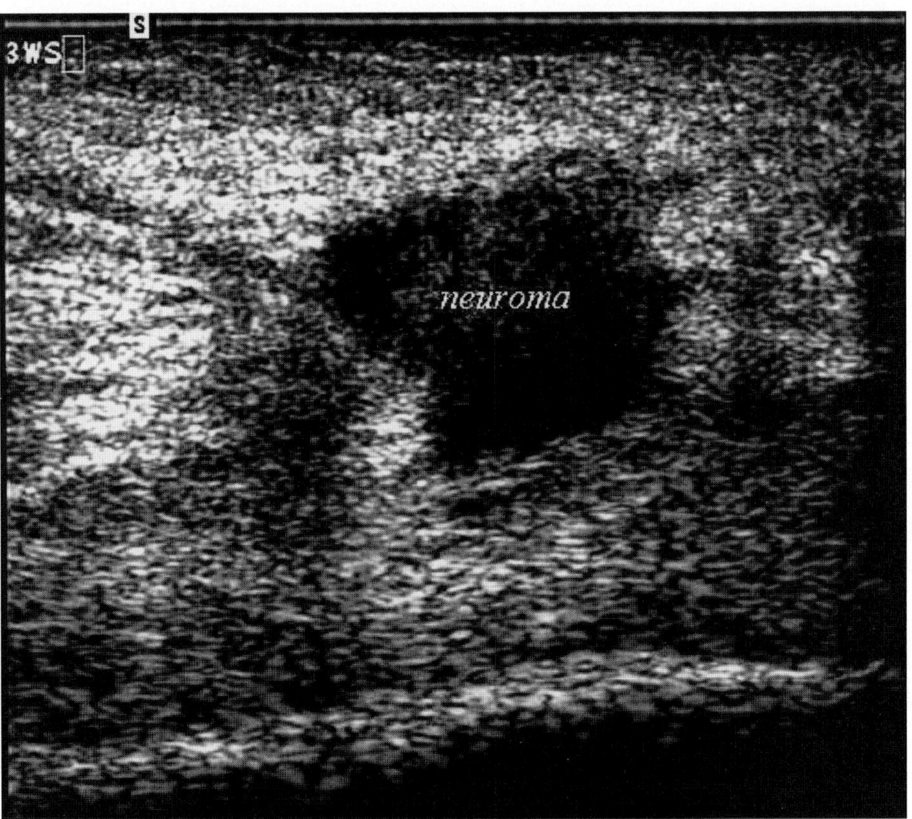

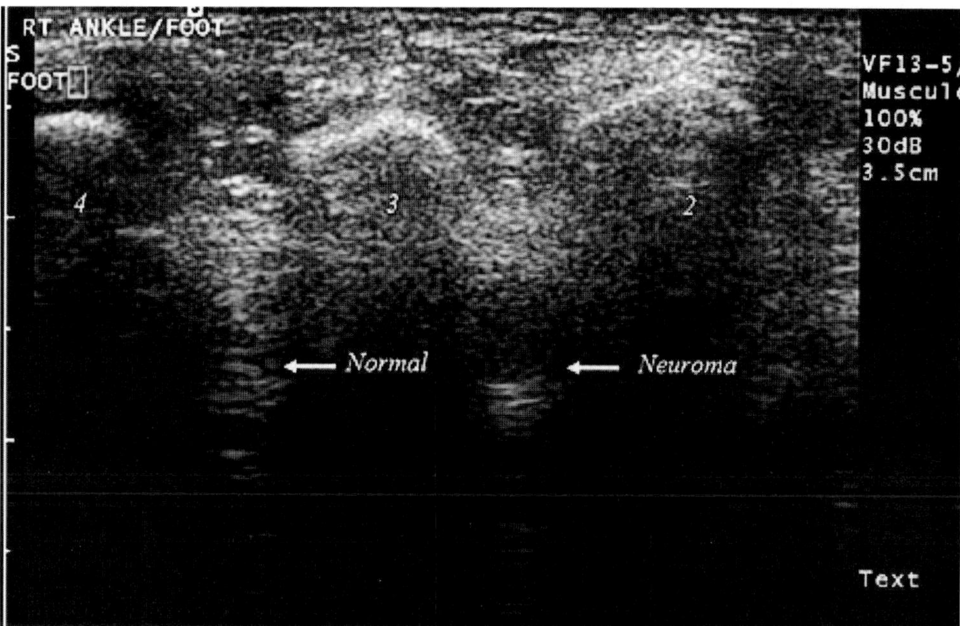

FIG. 2-5. Transverse image of the forefoot demonstrating a normal third web space (normal) and a second web space neuroma; note that the hyperechoic fat is replaced with a round, well-defined hypoechoic mass. The metatarsals are indicated (2, 3, and 4).

such as ganglion cysts (Fig. 2-9), adventitial bursae (Fig. 2-10), fibrolipomas, giant cell tumors, and primary (or secondary) malignancies. Fortunately, many of these are exceeding uncommon within the web spaces.

Synovitis and osteoarthritis of the metatarsophalangeal and interphalangeal joints can be diagnosed with ultrasound. For evaluation of the metatarsophalangeal and interphalangeal joints, a high-frequency linear probe is generally employed (Figs. 2-11 and 2-12). Normally, the superficial echogenic contours of the bones are smooth, and a uniform joint space with minimal, if any, fluid is identified (Figs. 2-13 and 2-14). In the setting of synovitis, the joint capsule is distended with fluid, soft tissue, or both, often of mixed echogenicity, and regional inflammatory changes can be demonstrated with power Doppler (Figs. 2-15 and 2-16). Frank erosions or discretely marginated cystlike changes of the juxtaarticular cortical surfaces can be seen, such as those in cases of gout or rheumatoid arthritis (Figs. 2-17 and 2-18). Given the superficial nature of the articulations of the forefoot, sonographic guidance for arthrocentesis or therapeutic injection can be easily performed (Fig. 2-19). Bunion deformities are treated effectively with ultrasound-guided injections. In our experience, patients have been content with the results of ultrasound-guided therapeutic injection, thereby often avoiding surgical intervention.

FIG. 2-4. Longitudinal ultrasound image of the third web space demonstrating a well-defined hypoechoic mass replacing the normally hyperechoic interdigital fat, consistent with a neuroma.

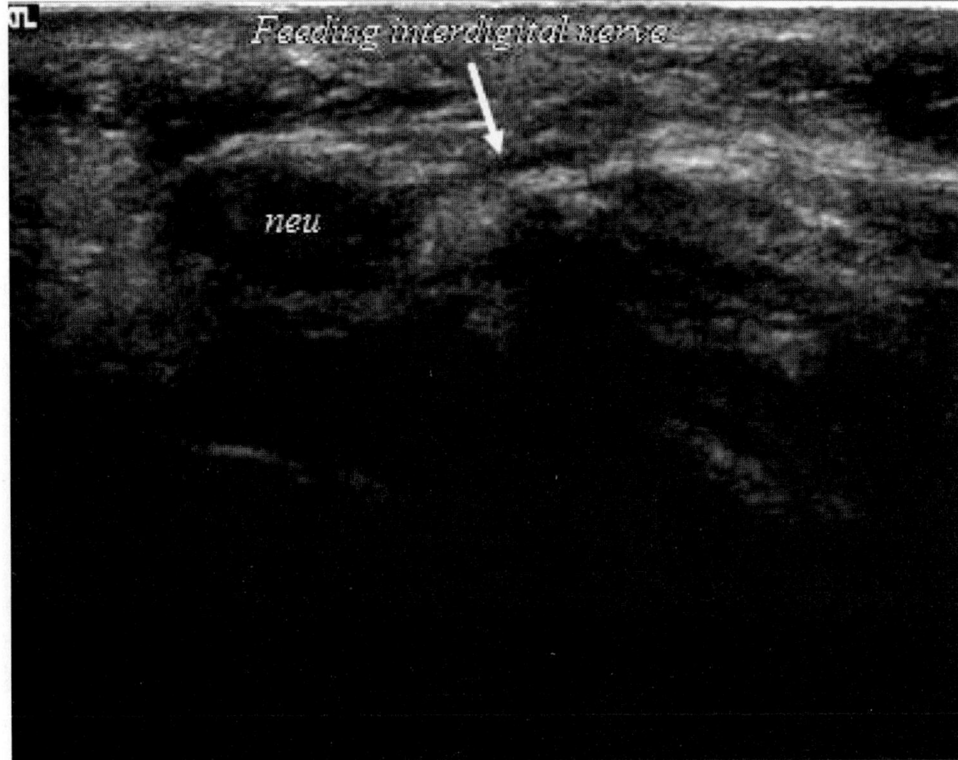

A

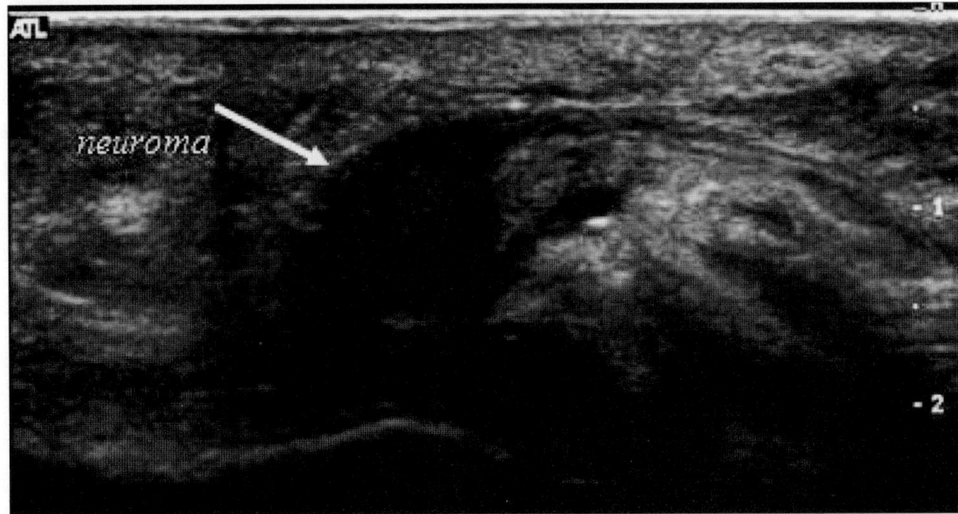

B

FIG. 2-6. A: Longitudinal image of the second web space demonstrating a neuroma (neu). Note the comet tail appearance of the proximal border of the neuroma, consistent with feeding interdigital nerve (*arrow*). **B:** Longitudinal ultrasound image in a different patient again demonstrating a tubular enlarged interdigital nerve associated with the second webspace neuroma. A small anechoic collection is seen to the right of the neuroma, corresponding to a small associated adventitial bursa.

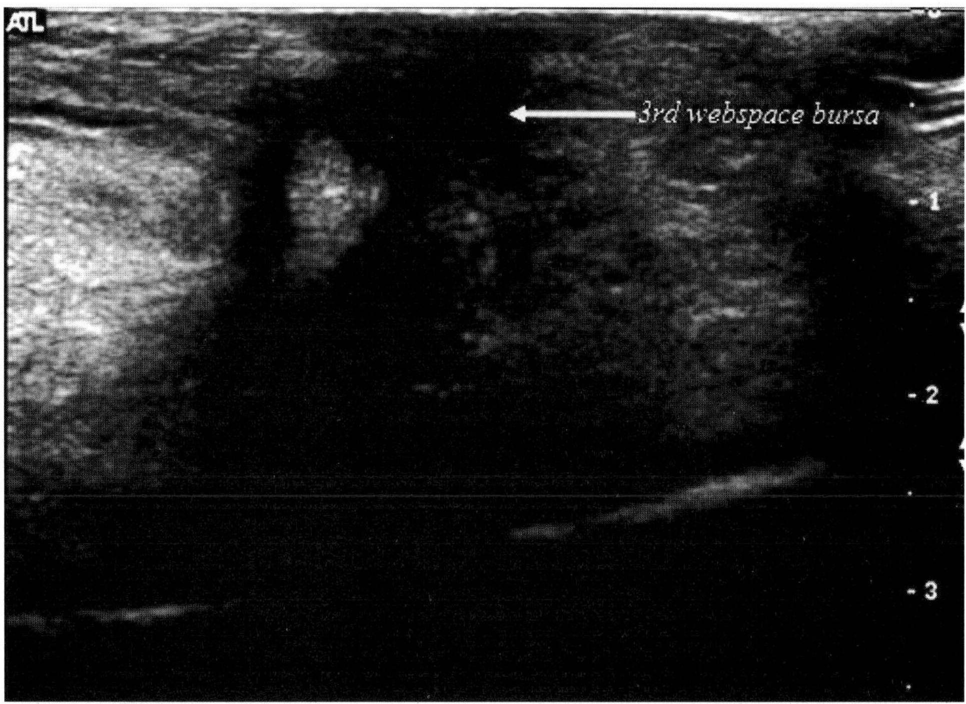

FIG. 2-7. Longitudinal ultrasound image of the third web space demonstrates an irregular hypoechoic collection that was compressible, consistent with an intermetatarsal bursa.

The margins of the bones of the forefoot are, in general, smooth and linear. Radio-occult fractures of the bones of the forefoot can be seen with sonography as focal offset or stepoff in the cortical surface (Fig. 2-20), often with regional periosteal hyperemia when power Doppler is applied. Adjacent subperiosteal fluid collections (hematomas) can also be identified.

Soft tissue impingement by indwelling hardware and screws, as well as secondary inflammatory changes, should be assessed (Figs. 2-21 and 2-22).

(Text continues on page 32)

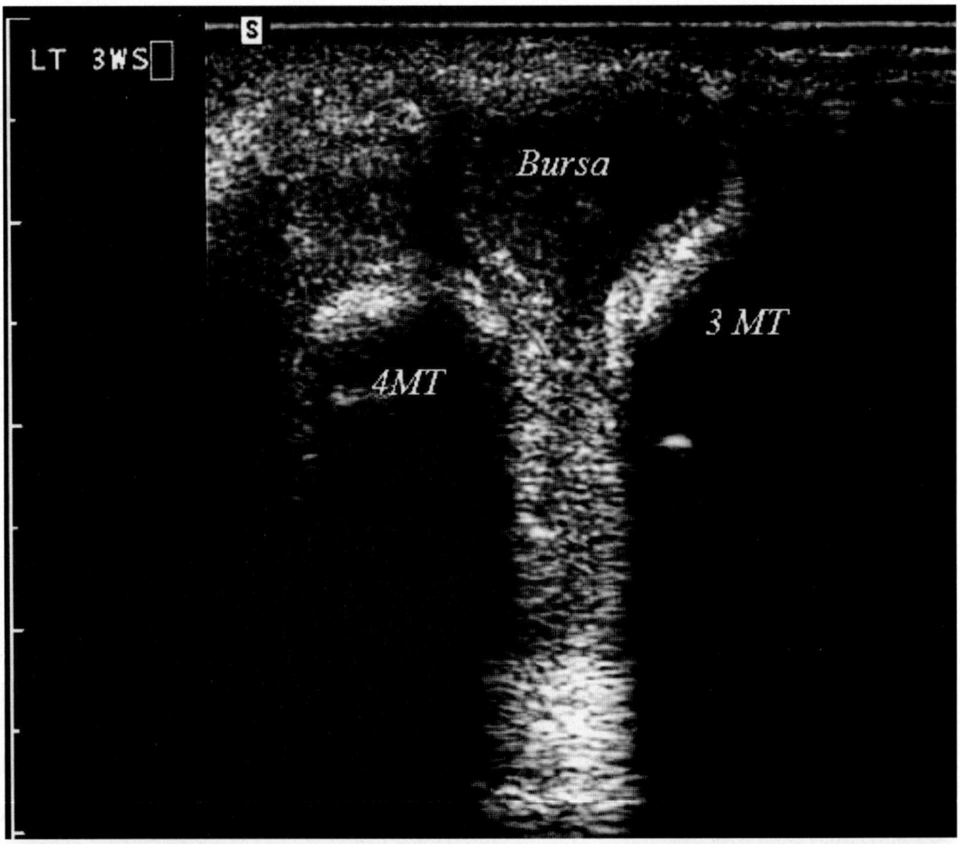

LT 3WS

Bursa

3 MT

4MT

A

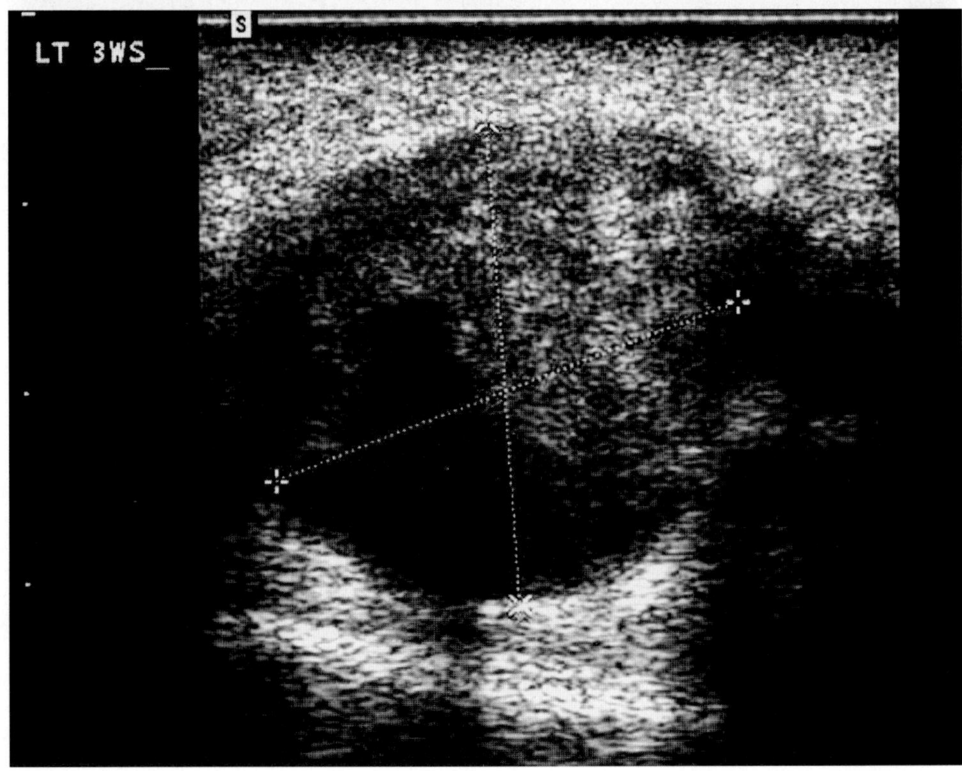

B

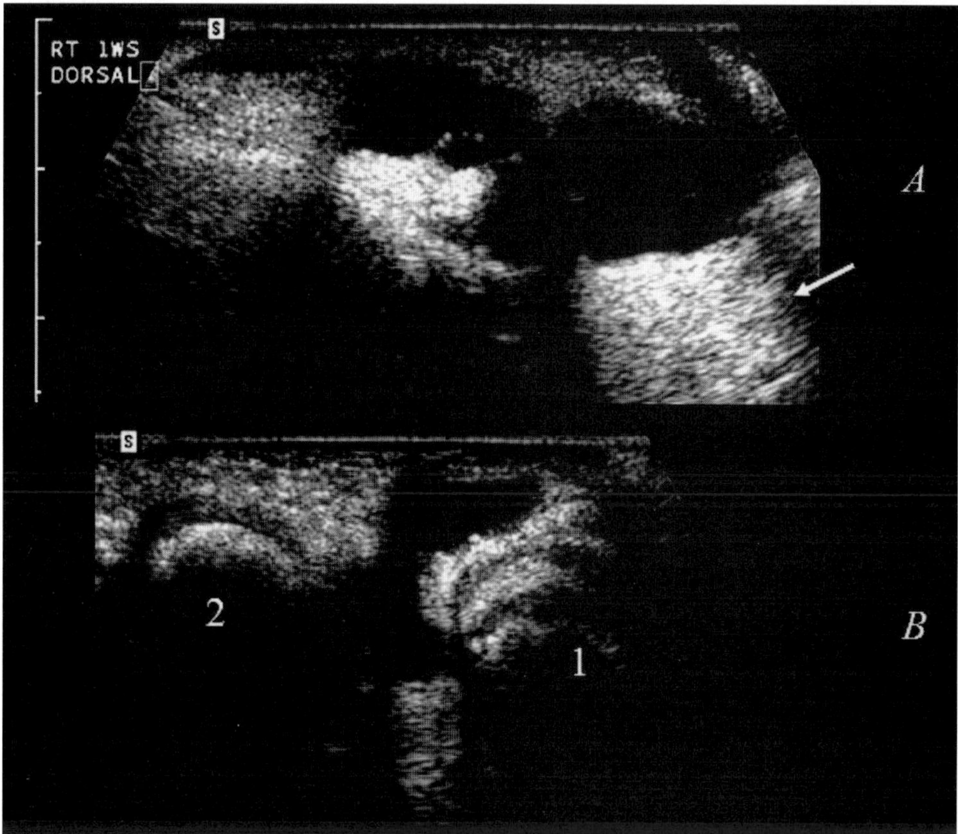

FIG. 2-9. A: Longitudinal sector image of the dorsal aspect of the forefoot at the level of the first webspace demonstrating a large complex ganglion cyst. Note the increased through-transmission typically seen with fluid-filled masses (*arrow*). **B:** Transverse view of the first web space demonstrating the relationship of the cyst to the first and second metatarsals (1 and 2, respectively). The cyst was noted to be hard and intimately associated with the joint capsule of the first metatarsophalangeal (MTP) joint, helping to distinguish it from a bursa.

FIG. 2-8. A: Transverse image at the level of the third and fourth metatarsal heads, seen in short axis (3MT and 4MT). The bones seen in short axis demonstrate strong echogenic superficial interfaces, with posterior acoustic shadowing. Note the complex hypoechoic material distending the third webspace consistent with an intermetatarsal bursa. **B:** Longitudinal sonogram over the dorsal aspect of the same patient better depicts the full extent (*calipers*) and complex nature of the bursa.

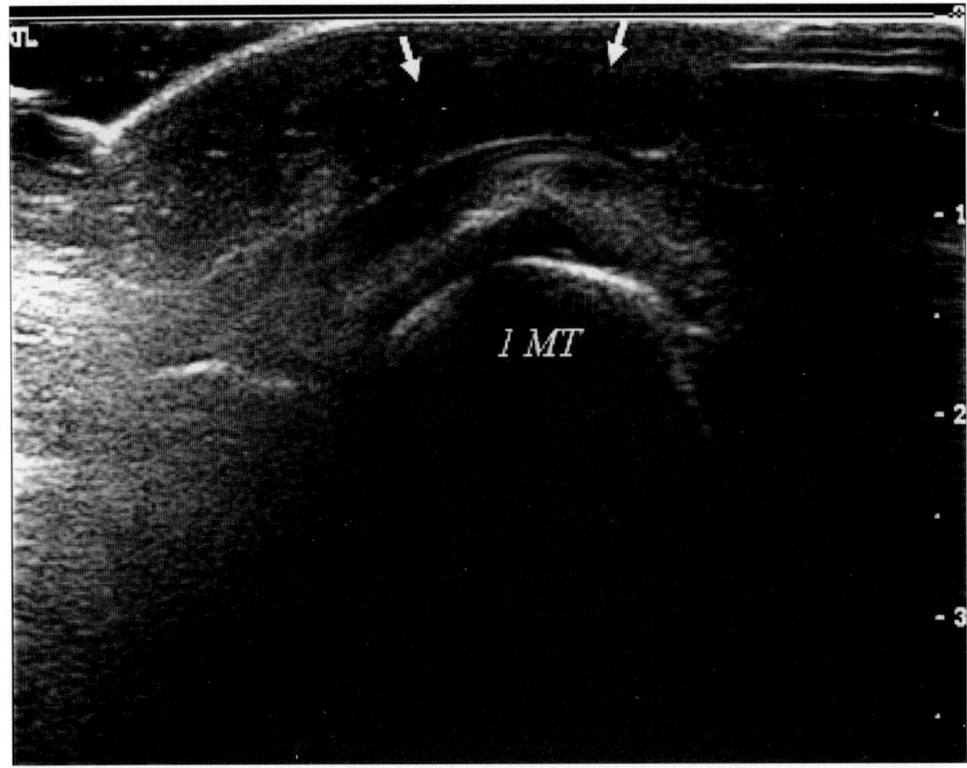

FIG. 2-10. Longitudinal ultrasound image along the plantar aspect of the foot at the level of the first metatarsal head demonstrates an encapsulated, mildly heterogeneous collection superficial to flexor hallucis longus tendon consistent with an adventitial bursa. The flexor hallucis longus tendon is immediately below the collection, and portions of the proximal phalanx are present to the left of the metatarsal head (1 MT).

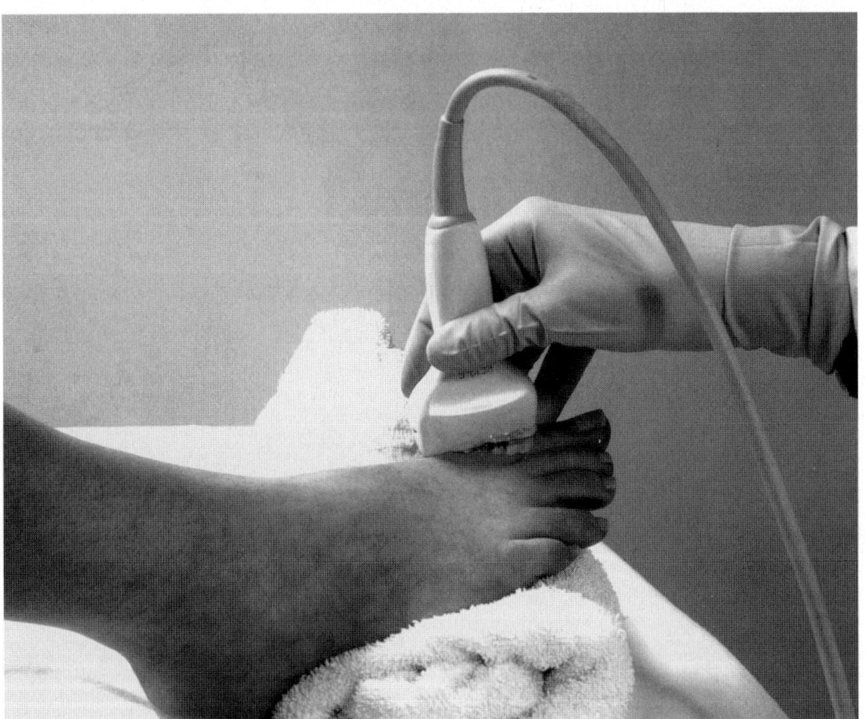

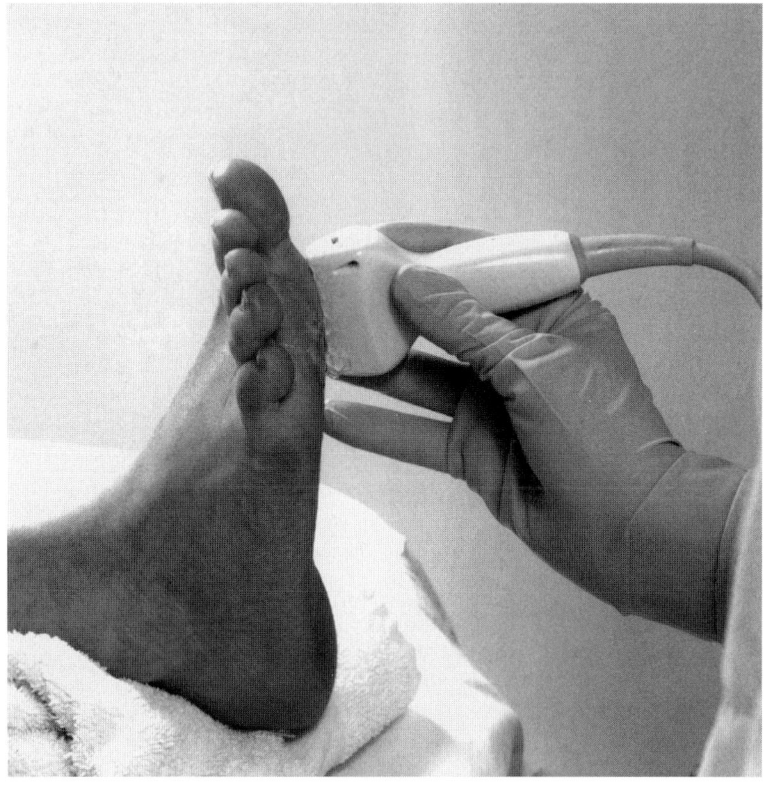

A

FIG. 2-12. A: The sesamoids and flexor hallucis longus tendon can be imaged from both a longitudinal and a transverse approach. For a longitudinal approach, as demonstrated here, the patient is supine and the foot dorsiflexed; the ultrasound probe is placed over the plantar margin of the first metatarsophalangeal (MTP) joint.

FIG. 2-12. *(Continued on next page)*

FIG. 2-11. Transducer positioning for imaging the first metatarsophalangeal (MTP) joint. Longitudinal images of the first MTP joint are obtained with the foot neutral or slightly plantarflexed, resting against a rolled towel or a bolster for support.

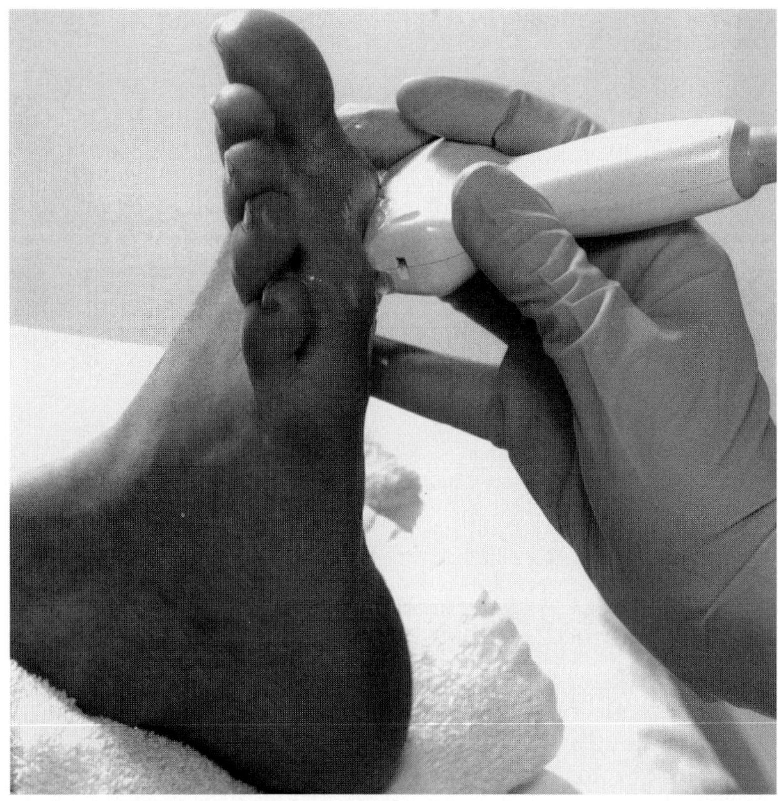

B

FIG. 2-12. B: Proper patient positioning for obtaining a transverse view of the sesamoids and distal flexor hallucis longus tendon.

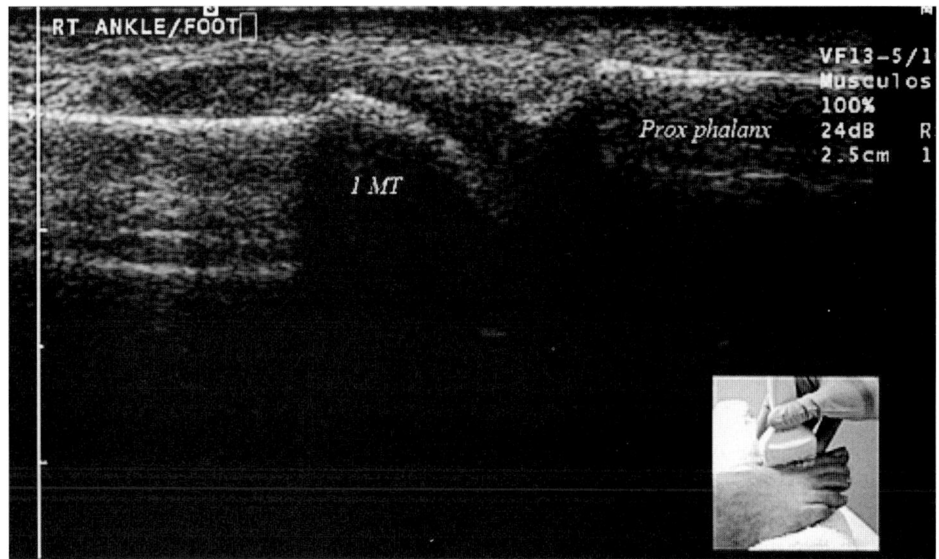

A

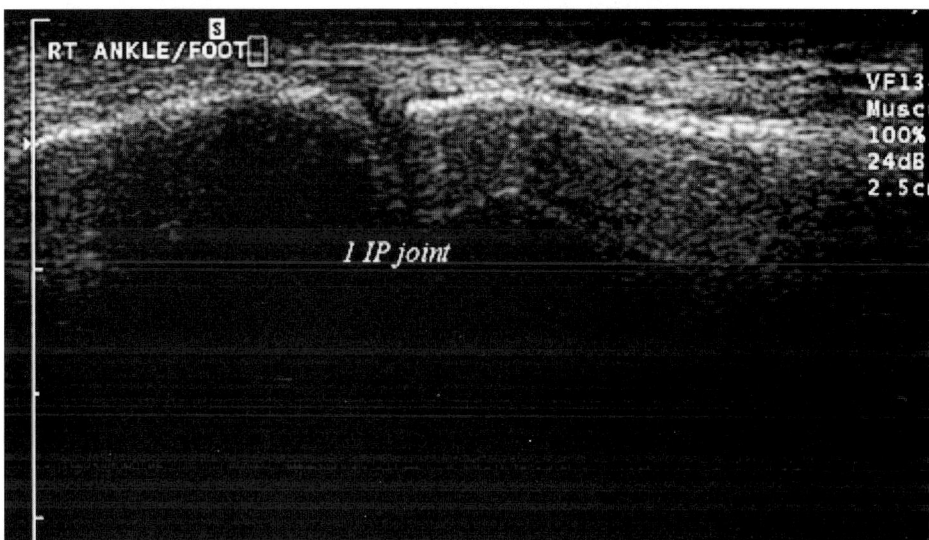

B

FIG. 2-13. A: Longitudinal image of the first metatarsophalangeal (MTP) joint. Cortical bone is seen as a sharp linear echogenic interface with posterior acoustic shadowing in contrast to the hypoechoic joint space. The joint appears as a discontinuity in the normally continuous cortical surface. The first metatarsal (1 MT) and proximal phalanx are indicated. **B:** Longitudinal image of the interphalangeal (IP) joint of the great toe. Cortical bone is seen as a sharp linear echogenic interface with posterior acoustic shadowing. The joint space is uniformly hypoechoic.

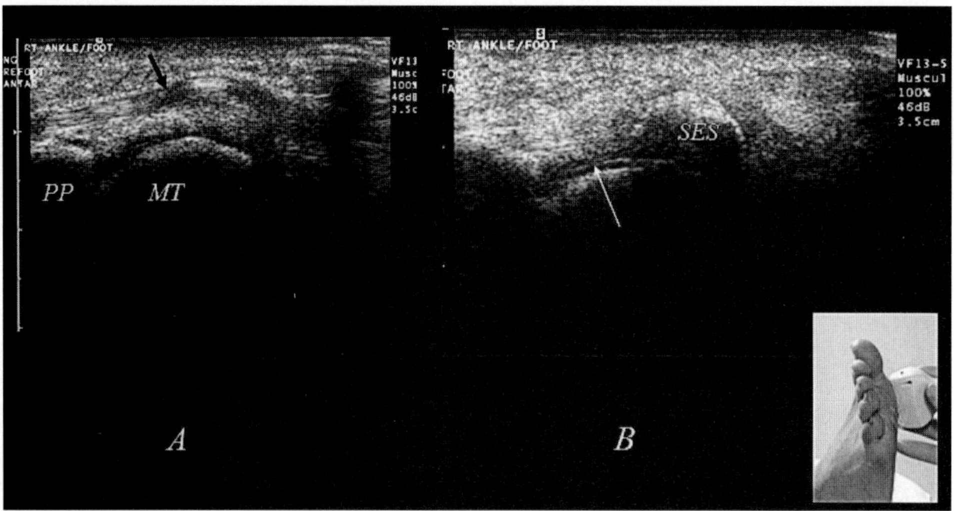

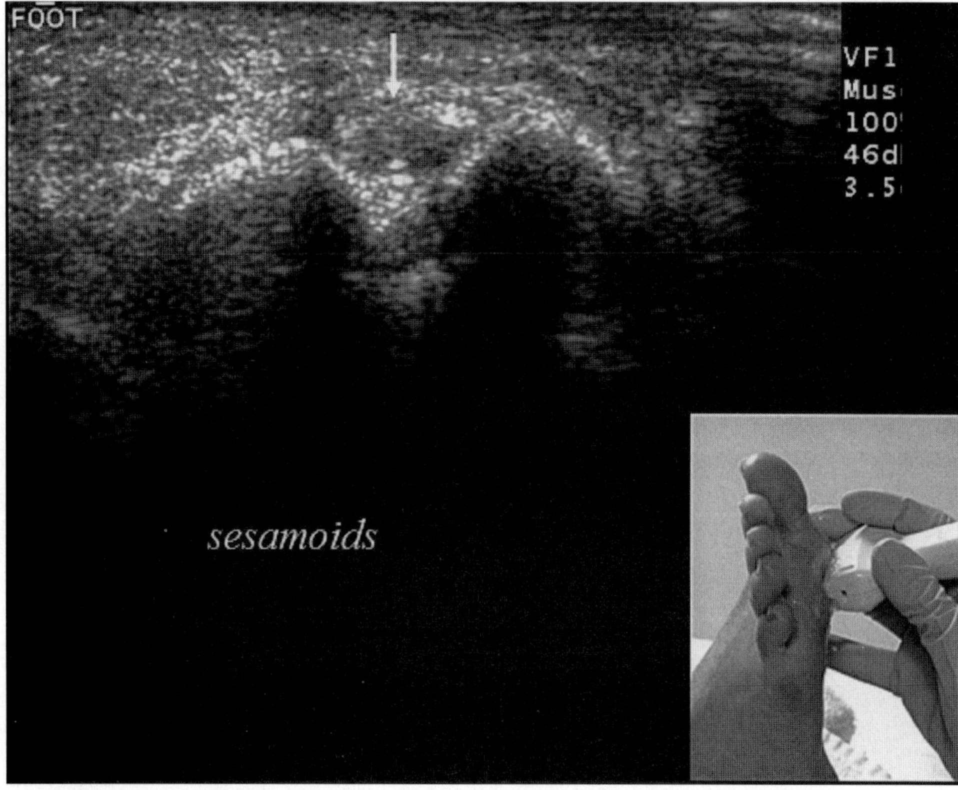

C

FIG. 2-14. Longitudinal images of the plantar aspect of the first metatarsophalangeal (MTP) joint at two slightly offset parasagittal planes. **A:** The first image on the **left** demonstrates the flexor hallucis longus tendon (*black arrow*). The first metatarsal and proximal phalanx (MT and PP, respectively) are indicated. **B:** The second image (transducer slightly more medial) demonstrates the medial sesamoid (SES). The normal uniformly hypoechoic articular cartilage over the first metatarsal head can also be seen (*long thin white arrow*). **C:** Transverse ultrasound image of the sesamoids. Note the normal, curvilinear sesamoids demonstrating posterior acoustic shadowing. The flexor hallucis longus tendon can be seen in cross section (*arrow*).

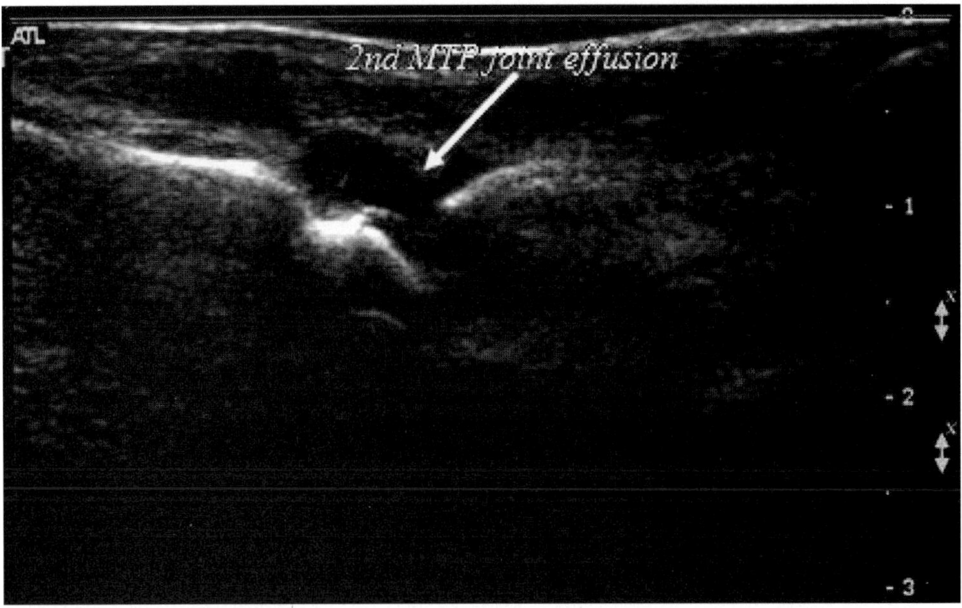

FIG. 2-15. Longitudinal ultrasound image of the second metatarsophalangeal (MTP) joint demonstrates a small effusion with thickening of the dorsal joint capsule (*white arrow*).

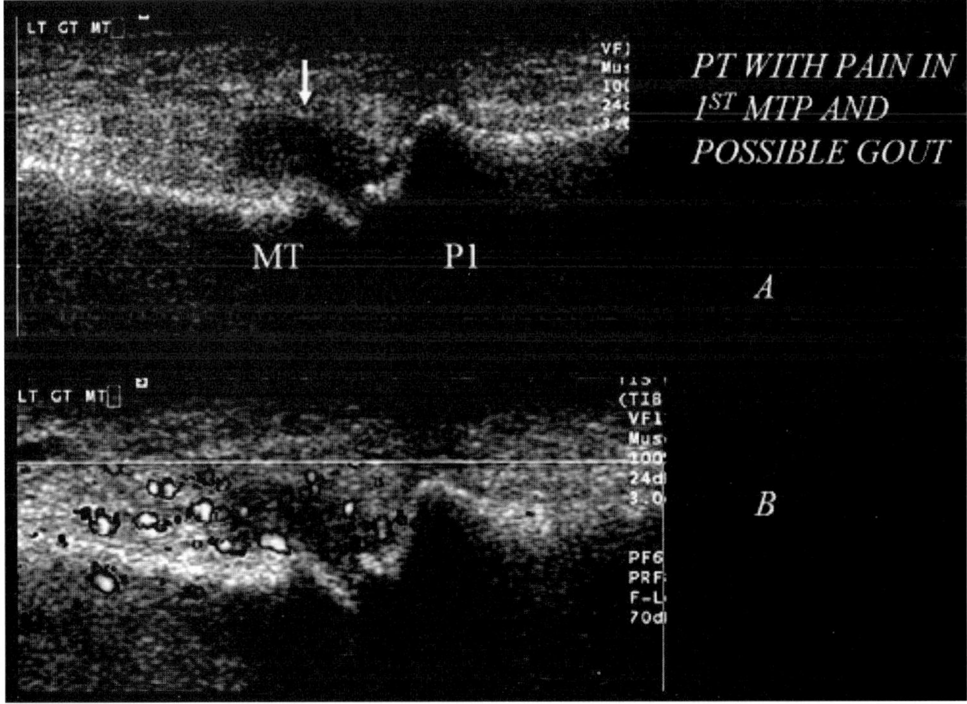

FIG. 2-16. A: Longitudinal view of the first metatarsophalangeal (MTP) joint in a patient with pain and swelling and clinical concern of gout. Hypoechoic debris is seen distending the joint space (*arrow*). The metatarsal head (MT) and proximal phalanx (P1) are labeled. **B:** There is marked regional hyperemia when power Doppler is applied, consistent with inflammation.

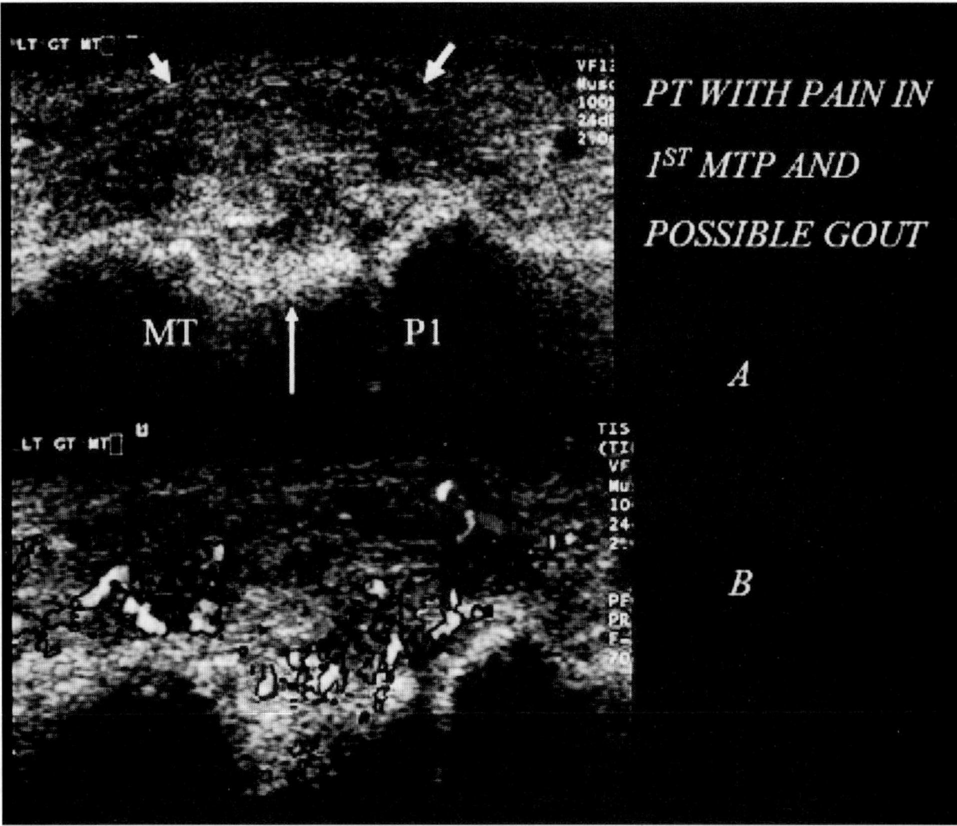

FIG. 2-17. A: Longitudinal image over the medial joint line of the first metatarsophalangeal (MTP) joint in the same patient as shown in Fig. 2–16 depicts cortical irregularity (*long arrow*) of the first metatarsal head (MT). A well-defined heterogeneous soft tissue mass (*short arrows*) abuts the cortical surface of the metatarsal head. **B:** Power Doppler imaging of the same area displays abnormal vascularity within the mass as well as adjacent to the cortical surface of the MTP joint. These features reflect the inflammatory nature of this tophaceous deposit.

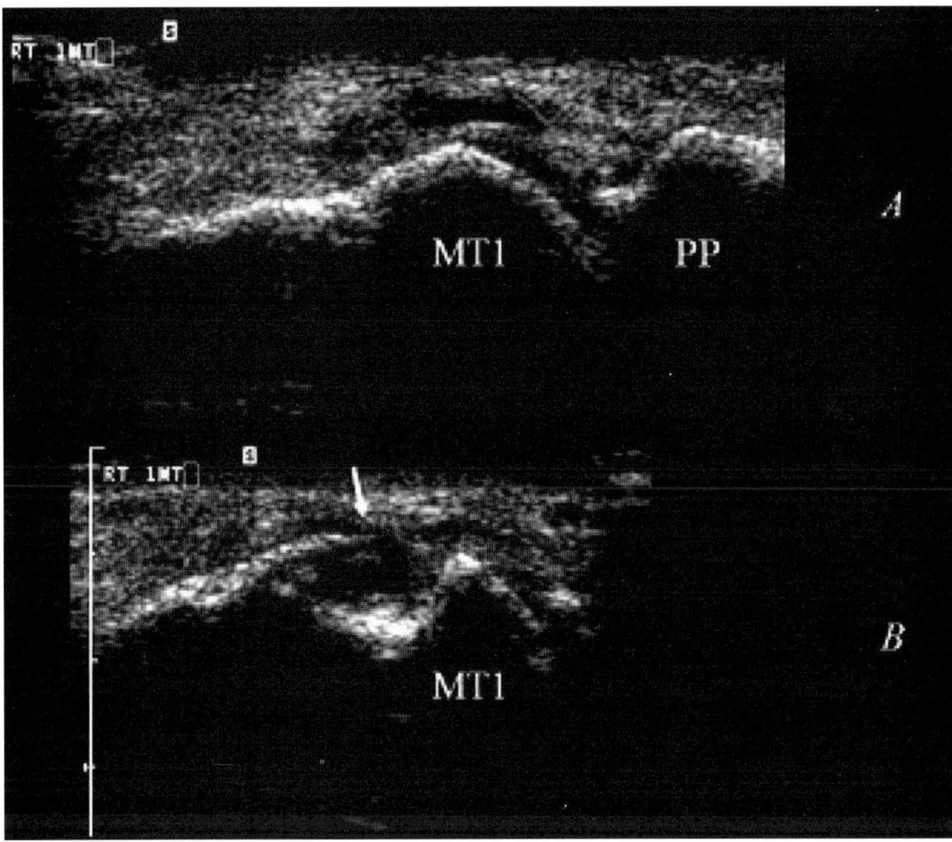

FIG. 2-18. A: Longitudinal image of the first metatarsophalangeal (MTP) joint in a patient with hallux valgus deformity demonstrating a small effusion. The first metatarsal (MT1) and proximal phalanx (PP) are labeled. **B:** Long axis view of the first MTP joint in the same patient, scanned along the medial joint line, demonstrates cystic change in the first metatarsal head (*arrow*).

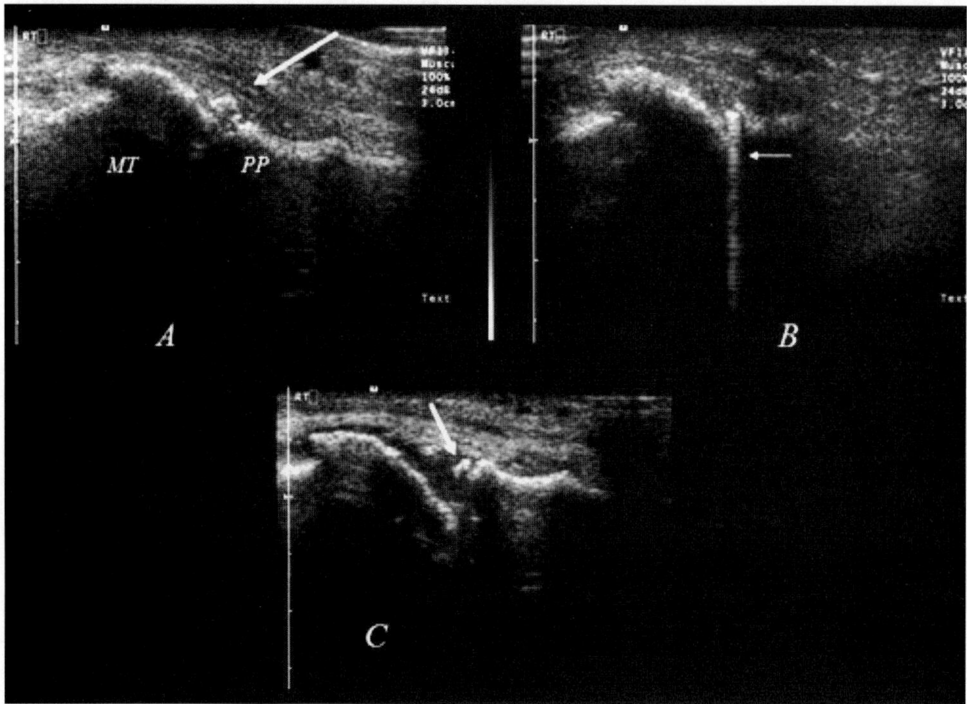

FIG. 2-19. A: Longitudinal ultrasound image of the first metatarsophalangeal (MTP) joint demonstrating moderate osteoarthritis. A small joint body is indicated (*arrow*). **B:** Ultrasound-guided placement of a 25-gauge needle within the first MTP joint displays the characteristic ring down artifact (*arrow*) produced by the needle, confirming its intraarticular position. **C:** After needle removal, the dorsal recess of the joint is distended by a steroid-anesthetic mixture, and the joint body (*arrow*) is floating.

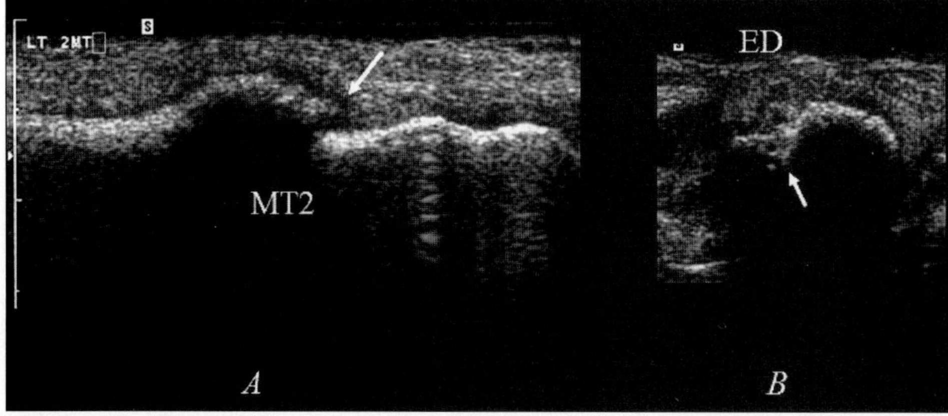

FIG. 2-20. Longitudinal **(A)** and short axis **(B)** views of the second metatarsal demonstrating focal cortical irregularity (*arrow*) of the second metatarsal consistent with a fracture. Radiographs were negative 1 month earlier, and ultrasound was requested because the patient was having persistent second metatarsal pain. The extensor digitorum longus tendon (ED) is indicated.

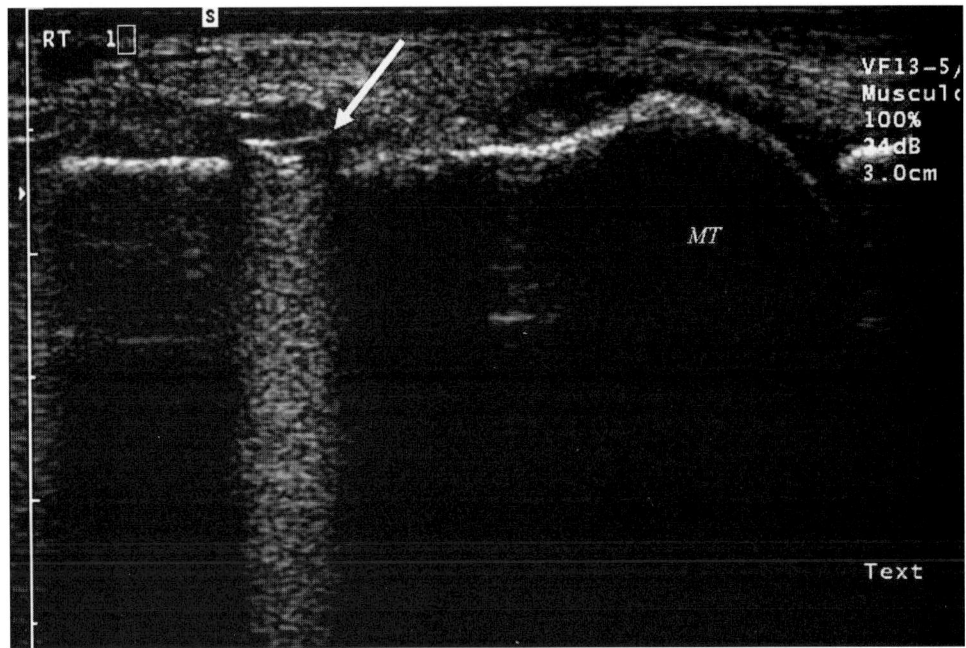

FIG. 2-21. Longitudinal ultrasound image at the level of the first metatarsal after osteotomy for hallux valgus demonstrates fixation screw, which appears as a linear surface with strong posterior reverberation (*arrow*).

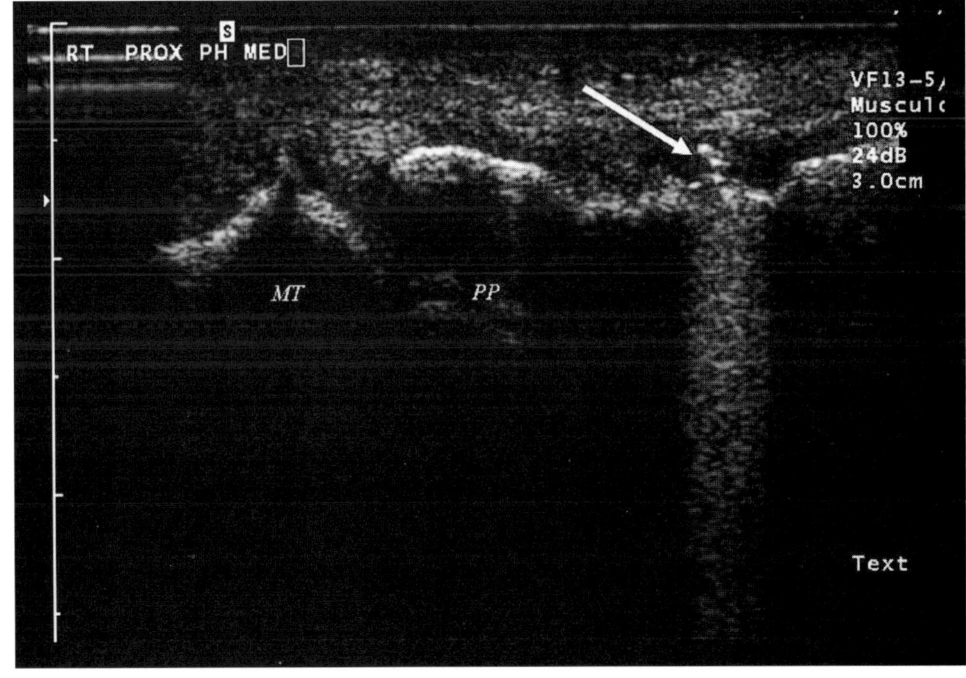

FIG. 2-22. A: Longitudinal image at the level of the metatarsophalangeal (MTP) joint of the first ray after osteotomy for hallux valgus shows a screw with characteristic metallic artifact (*arrow*) perforating the cortex of the proximal phalanx.

FIG. 2-22. *(Continued on next page)*

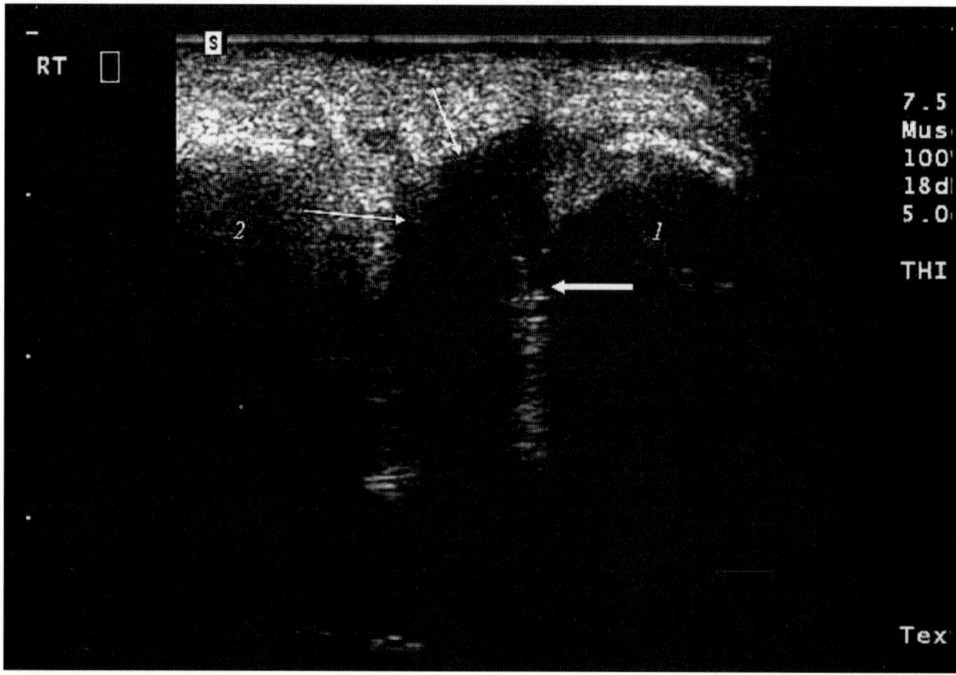

B

FIG. 2-22. B: A second screw was present within the lateral joint (*thick arrow*), resulting in a secondary inflammatory reaction. The latter appears as hypoechoic soft tissue (*thin arrows*) surrounding the screw and contiguous with the lateral joint margin.

REFERENCES

1. Iagnocco A, Coari G, Palombi G, et al. Sonography in the study of metatarsalgia. *J Rheumatol* 2001;28: 1338–1340.
2. Quinn TJ, Jacobson JA, Craig JG, et al. Sonography of Morton's neuromas. *AJR Am J Roentgenol* 2000;174 (6):1723–1728.
3. Morscher E, Ulrich J, Dick W. Morton's intermetatarsal neuroma: morphology and histological substrate. *Foot Ankle Int* 2000;21(7):558–562.
4. Read JW, Noakes JB, Kerr D, et al. Morton's metatarsalgia: sonographic findings and correlated histopathology. *Foot Ankle Int* 1999;20(3):153–161.
5. Fessell DP, van Holsbeeck MT. Foot and ankle sonography. *Radiol Clin North Am* 1999;37(4):831–858.
6. Levine SE, Myerson MS, Shapiro PP, et al. Ultrasonographic diagnosis of recurrence after excision of an interdigital neuroma. *Foot Ankle Int* 1998;19(2):79–84.

3

Midfoot

Midfoot pathology that can be evaluated with sonography includes soft tissue ganglia (Fig. 3-1), bursae (Fig. 3-2) and other soft tissue masses, tendinosis (Fig. 3-3), tendon tears (Fig. 3-4), tenosynovitis (Fig. 3-5), and midfoot arthrosis (Fig. 3-6). In the setting of trauma, ligamentous injury and subtle cortical stepoff may be evident (Fig. 3-7), although ultrasound should never be considered a replacement for conventional radiography.

Soft tissue ganglia are seen as discrete, encapsulated, hypoechoic masses, often in close proximity to an arthritic joint (1,2) (Fig. 3-1). There is usually little, if any, regional hyperemia on Doppler imaging. Posterior acoustic enhancement may be identified as well as edge artifact, although the posterior margin may be obscured by cortical bone. The material within the ganglia is often very viscous, and sonographically guided aspiration of the cysts, even with a large-gauge needle, can yield little or no fluid. Injection of the cysts, however, with corticosteroids usually results in significant pain relief and shrinkage of the cysts.

The dorsal compartment tendons as they cross the midfoot (tibialis anterior, extensor hallucis longus, and extensor digitorum longus) can all be clearly visualized using either a medium- or high-frequency linear transducer (Fig. 3-8). Normally, the tendons are seen as tightly packed, linear, echogenic bands displaying a characteristic fibrillar architecture (3) (Fig. 3-9). Even a small amount of fluid in the tendon sheaths can be identified using high frequency transducers, and therefore, the tendon sheaths can easily be accessed percutaneously using sonographic guidance.

All of the articulations of the midfoot can be identified during routine sonographic evaluation (Fig. 3-10). Normally, the superficial, echogenic contours of the bones of the midfoot are smooth and uniform, with joint spaces seen as discontinuities between bones with a thin echogenic dorsal capsule crossing the articular margins (Fig. 3-11). In the presence of osteoarthritis, the smoothly marginated joint margins are replaced by dorsal osteophytes, identified as exophytic echogenic projections along the dorsal margin of the midfoot (Figs. 3-2 and 3-6.). The dorsal capsule is frequently hypertrophied and contains mixed echogenic debris, consistent with synovitis (Fig. 3-12).

The presence of indwelling orthopaedic hardware does not preclude sonographic evaluation of the overlying soft tissues (Fig. 3-4). The presence of plate and screw fixation, needles, or other instrumentation is characterized by echogenic margins with strong posterior reverberation artifact. Doppler imaging can further delineate active inflammation and neurovascular structures. As in the forefoot, radiographically occult fractures may be evident on sonography. Cuboid fractures, for example, often secondary to inversion injury, are often missed on standard radiographic views. Sonography clearly demonstrates the presence of small stepoffs along the cuboid bone margin.

(Text continues on page 40)

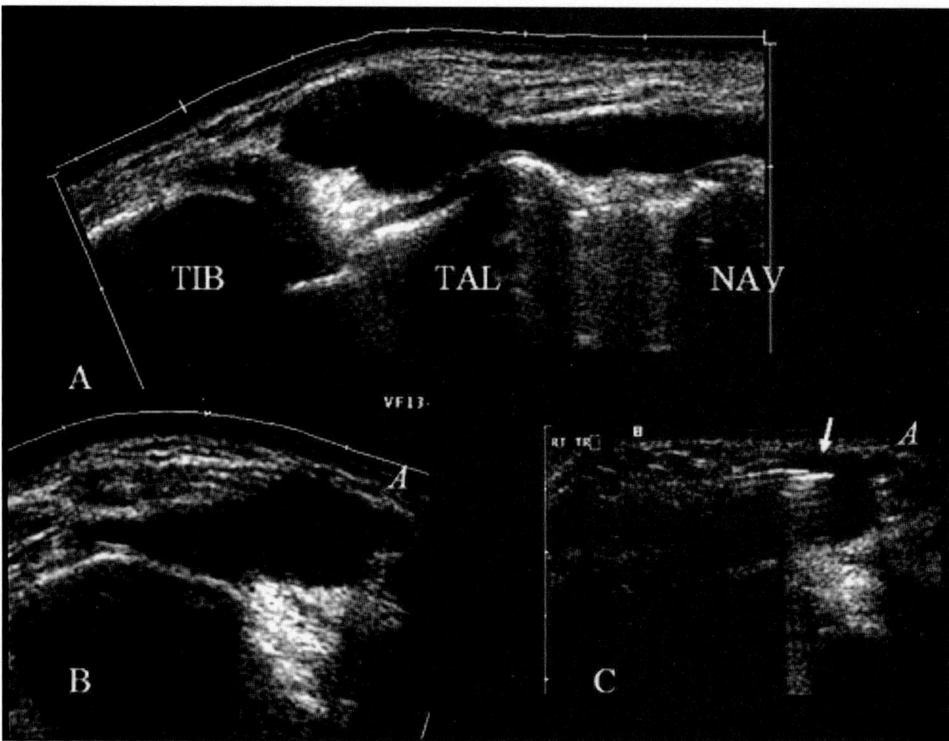

FIG. 3-1. Three images of the dorsum of the midfoot demonstrating a large ganglion cyst arising from the talonavicular joint capsule. Longitudinal **(A)** and transverse **(B)** extended field of view images demonstrate the relationship of the cyst to the bones of the midfoot: tibia (tib), talus (tal) and navicular (nav). The last image **(C)** is a short axis view demonstrating a needle (*arrow*) entering the cyst for therapeutic aspiration and injection.

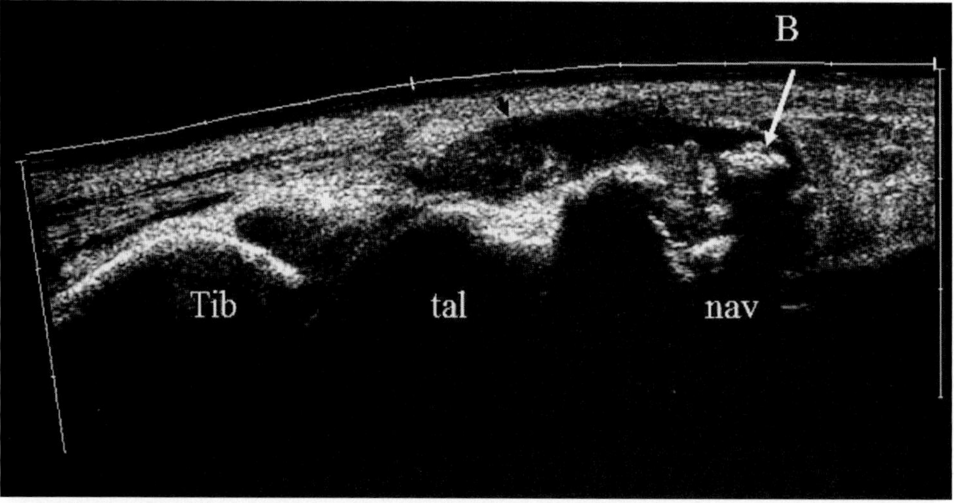

FIG. 3-2. Longitudinal extended field of view image demonstrating a complex synovial cyst (*arrowheads*) arising from an arthritic talonavicular joint; talus (tal) and navicular (nav) are indicated. Dorsal osteophytosis is seen arising from the navicular as well as an osteochrondral body (B) within the cyst. The tibia is also indicated (Tib) for reference. Distention of the tibiotalar joint by an effusion is evident.

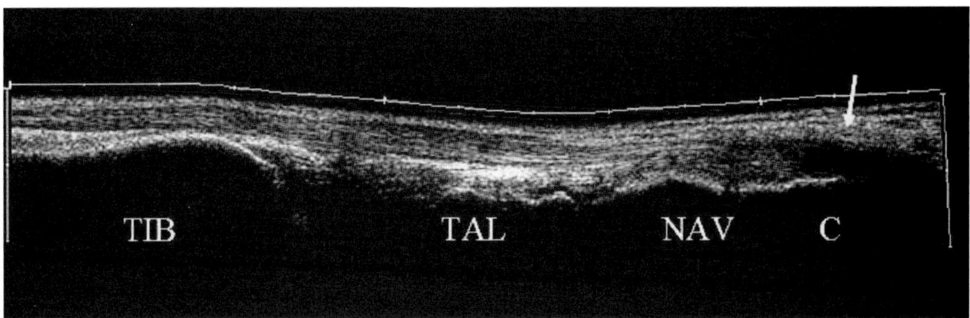

FIG. 3-3. Longitudinal extended field of view image of the midfoot demonstrating insertional tendinosis of the tibialis anterior tendon. Note the decreased echogenicity of the tendon at the insertion (*arrow*) onto the medial cuneiform. The tibia (TIB), talus (TAL), navicular (NAV), and medial cuneiform (C) are indicated.

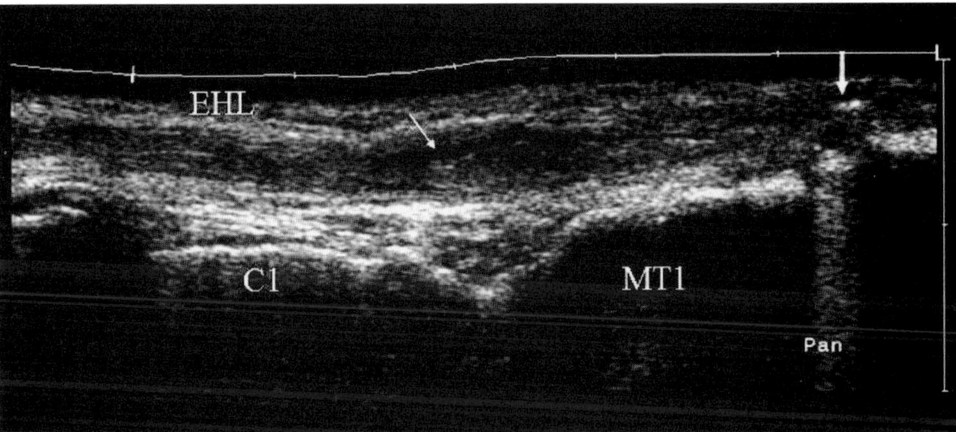

FIG. 3-4. Longitudinal extended field of view image in a patient with foot pain after first metatarsal osteotomy. Note the moderate extensor hallucis longus tendinosis with thickening, decreased echogenicity, and a split in the tendon (*thin arrow*). Distally, one can see a screw head in the first metatarsal (MT1) backing out of the bone and impinging the distal aspect of the tendon (*thick white arrow*). The medial cuneiform (C1) is indicated for reference.

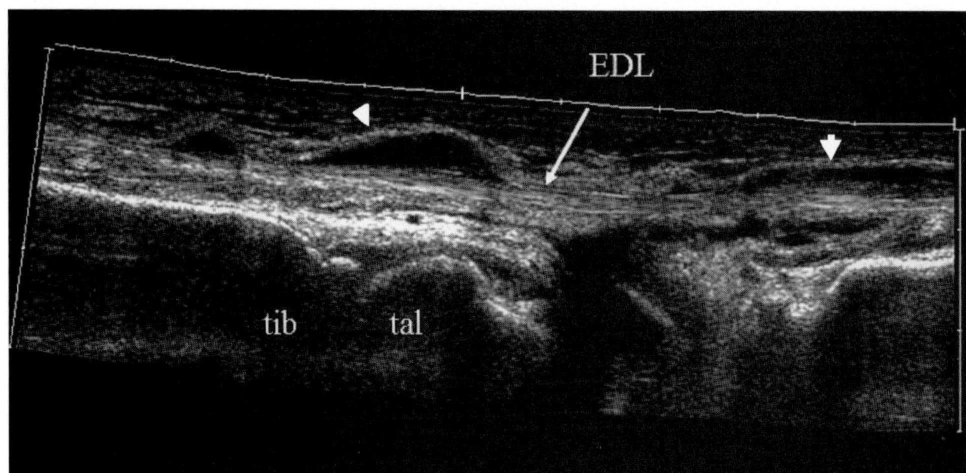

FIG. 3-5. Longitudinal extended field of view image demonstrating mild extensor digitorum longus (EDL) tendinosis with a loculated tendon sheath effusion (*white arrowheads*). The tibia (tib) and talus (tal) are indicated for reference. A small tibiotalar joint effusion is present.

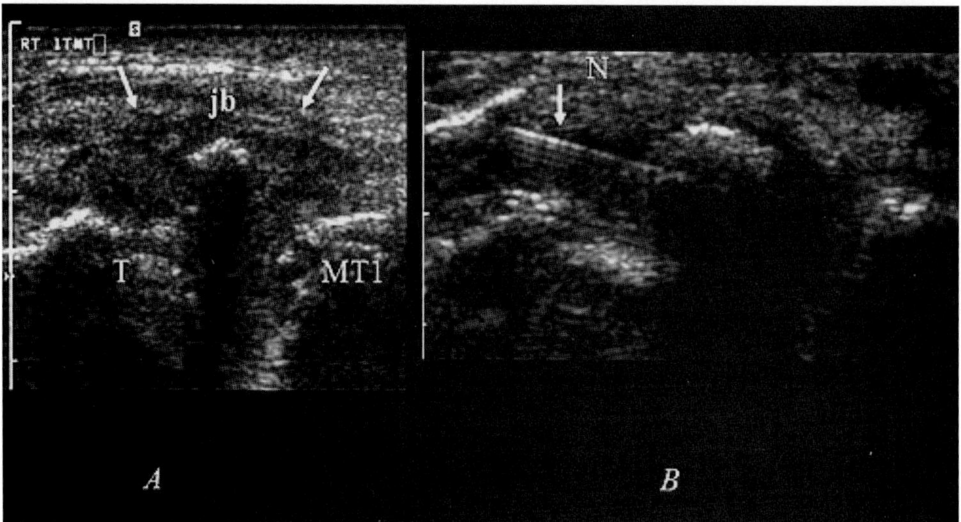

FIG. 3-6. Although plain radiographs allow assessment of bony abnormalities in patients with midfoot arthrosis, ultrasound provides additional information regarding capsular distention, the presence of synovial proliferation or joint fluid, and the presence of intraarticular bodies. **A:** In this case, the first tarsometatarsal joint is distended by complex soft tissue (*arrows*), which demonstrated marked hyperemia on power Doppler imaging (not shown). A small joint body (jb) is present, which could potentially interfere with guided joint injection. Note that the joint margins are irregular and distracted. **B:** In this short axis view, a 25-gauge needle (N) is positioned below the joint body, using ultrasound guidance, for purposes of therapeutic injection.

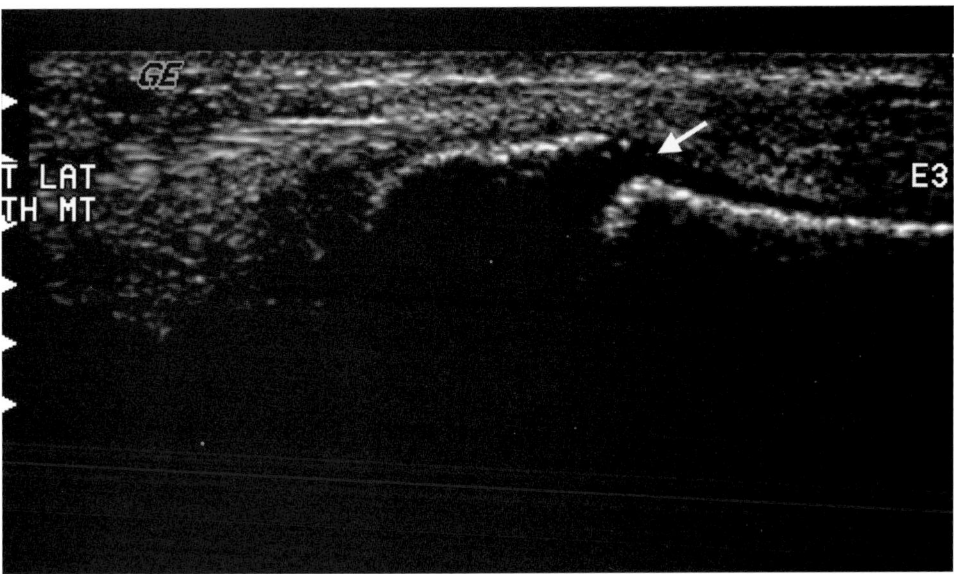

FIG. 3-7. Patient with lateral midfoot pain following an inversion injury. A cortical stepoff and subperiosteal hematoma are evident (*arrow*) at the site of a minimally displaced fracture of the base of the fifth metatarsal. A minimally displaced fracture was confirmed radiographically (not shown).

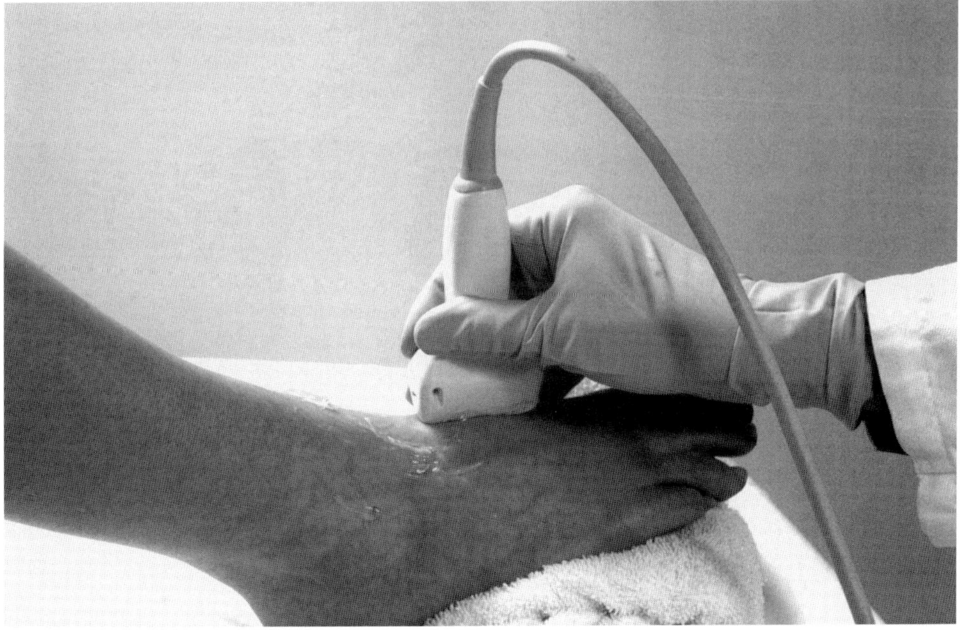

FIG. 3-8. Proper transducer positioning for imaging the tibialis anterior tendon in long axis at the level of the midfoot. The midfoot articulations are also best examined in this plane while continuously sweeping the transducer across the foot.

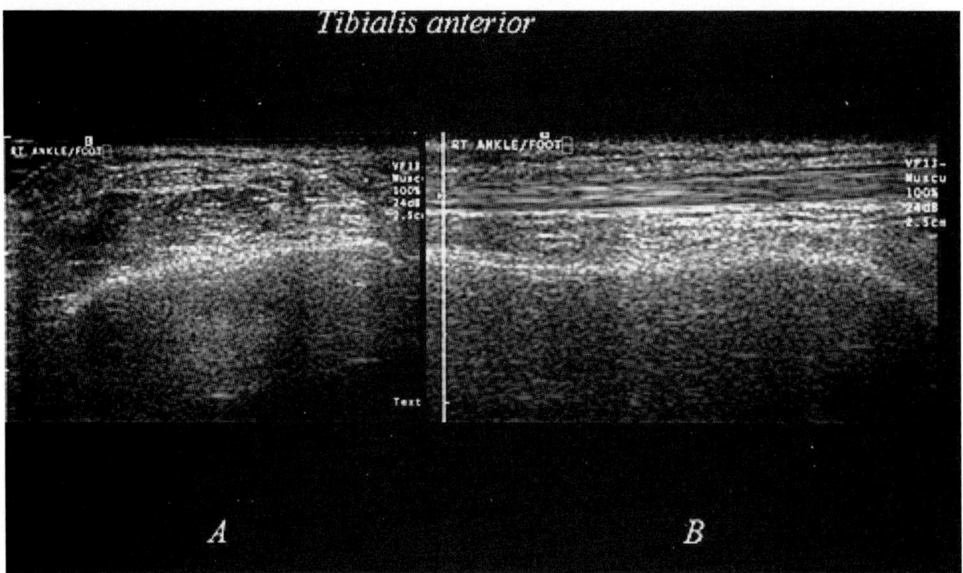

FIG. 3-9. Short axis **(A)** and long axis **(B)** views of the tibialis anterior tendon at level of the midfoot show a typical compact echogenic and fibrillar tendon morphology. The latter is best appreciated on the long axis view (**right**).

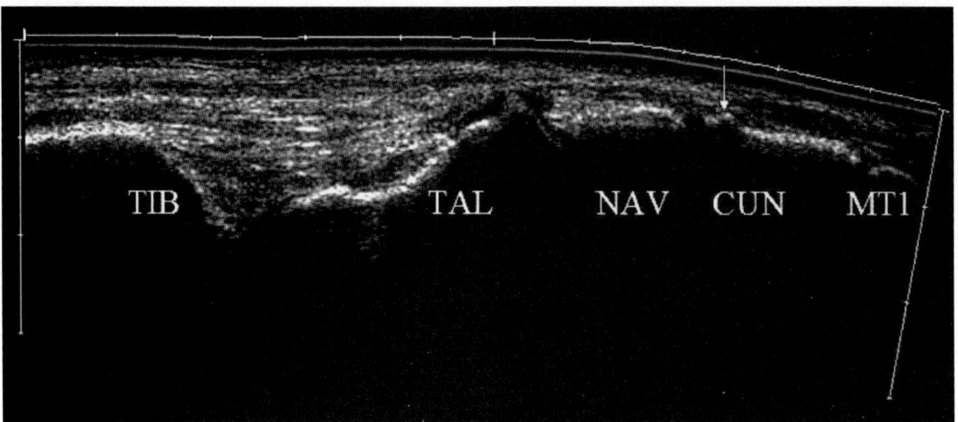

FIG. 3-10. Longitudinal extended field of view image demonstrating the relationship of the bones of the midfoot; the tibia (TIB), talus (TAL), navicular (NAV), medial cuneiform (CUN), and first metatarsal (MT1) are indicated. A small osteophyte is seen at the dorsal aspect of the medial cuneiform (*arrow*). Note the normally echogenic triangular fat pad at the tibiotalar joint. Displacement of the fat pad by fluid or other soft tissue is indicative of intraarticular pathology.

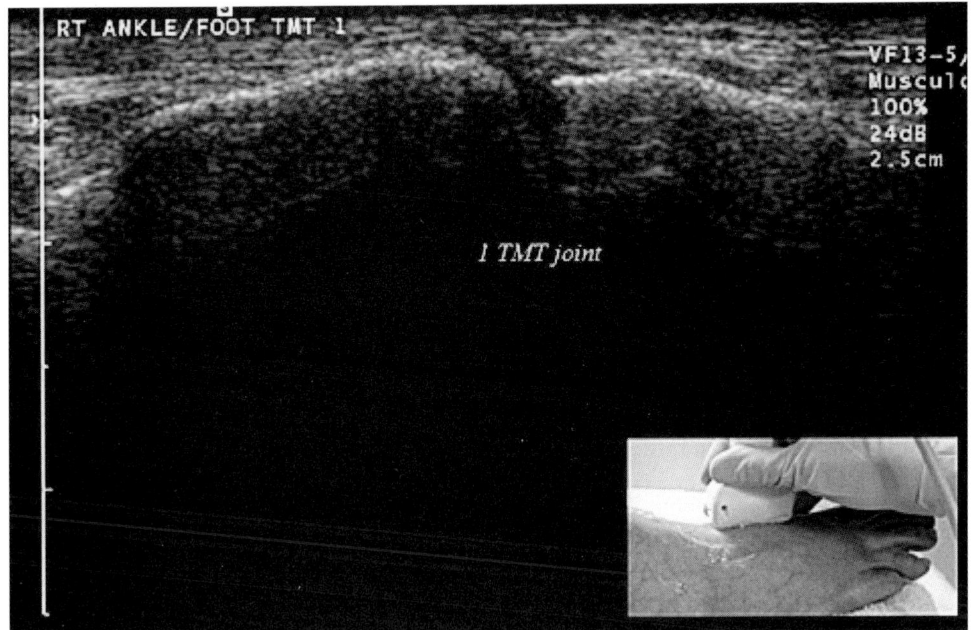

FIG. 3-11. Normal longitudinal image of the first tarsometatarsal joint. The joint space is evident as a discontinuity of the otherwise continuous cortical echo, separated by triangular echogenic fat. The joint capsule appears as a thin echogenic band along the superficial margin of the joint. Normally, as in this case, the capsule cannot be easily distinguished from the overlying soft tissues.

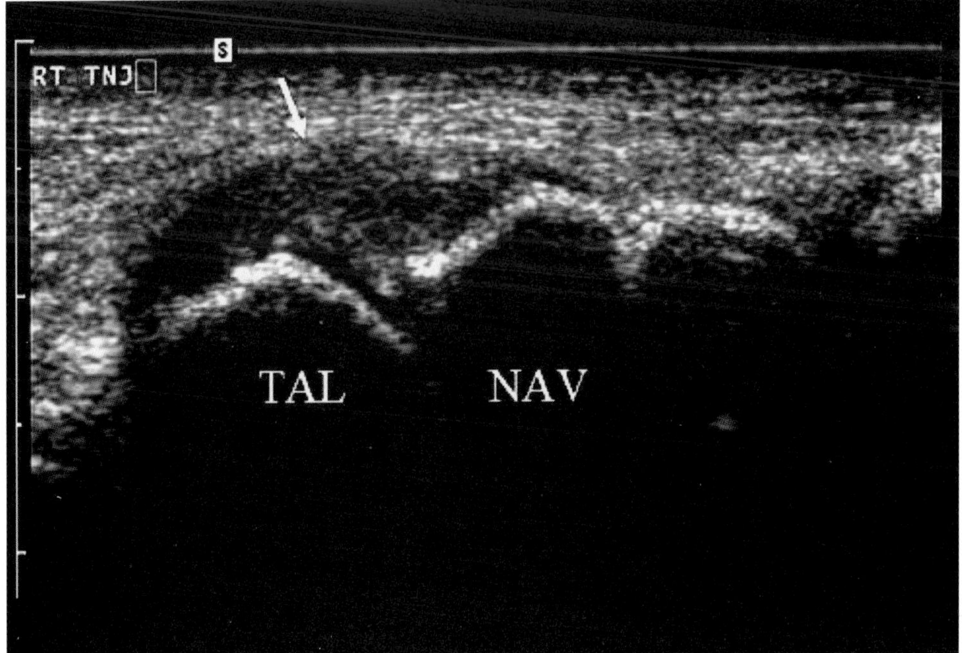

FIG. 3-12. Longitudinal ultrasound image of the talonavicular joint demonstrating hypoechoic soft tissue arising from the joint space consistent with a distended joint capsule (*arrow*) in a patient with pyrophosphate arthropathy. The talus (TAL) and navicular (NAV) are indicated.

REFERENCES

1. Ortega R, Fessell DP, Jacobson JA, et al. Sonography of ankle ganglia with pathologic correlation in 10 pediatric and adult patients. *AJR Am J Roentgenol* 2002;178:1445–1449.
2. Pham H, Fessell DP, Femino JE, et al. Sonography and MR imaging of selected benign masses in the ankle and foot. *AJR Am J Roentgenol* 2003;180:99–107.
3. Fessell DP, van Holsbeeck MT. Foot and ankle sonography. *Radiol Clin North Am* 1999;37(4):831–858.

4

Tendons and Ligaments about the Ankle

Tendons crossing the ankle can be divided into three compartments: the lateral compartment (peroneus brevis and longus), the anterior compartment (tibialis anterior, extensor hallucis longus, extensor digitorum longus), and the medial compartment (posterior tibial tendon, flexor digitorum longus, and flexor hallucis longus). All of these tendons, associated ligaments, and neurovascular structures, can be visualized with sonography.

In general, a high-frequency (13 MHz) linear transducer is employed. The lateral ankle tendons are seen to best advantage if the patient rests on the contralateral hip, with the lateral aspect of the ankle horizontal to the examining table (Fig. 4-1). The foot can be draped over several towels, which elevates the foot and allows gravity to pull the forefoot toward the floor, resulting in a smooth imaging surface around the lateral malleolus. Structures that can be readily examined include the peroneus longus and brevis tendons (Fig. 4-2), anterior talofibular and calcaneofibular ligaments (Fig. 4-3), and lateral gutter and adjacent cortical surfaces.

A similar approach can be used for examining the medial tendons, with the patient lying on the ipsilateral hip (Fig. 4-4). The medial compartment structures that should be examined include the posterior tibial tendon, flexor digitorum longus and flexor hallucis longus tendons, and intervening neurovascular bundle (for possible masses) (Figs. 4-5 to 4-7; see also Chapter 1). The deltoid ligament can also be examined with the patient in this position (Fig. 4-8).

The extensor tendons can be imaged with the patient supine, knee flexed, and foot flat on the imaging table, with the ultrasound probe in a direct anterior approach (Fig. 4-9). These include the tibialis anterior, extensor hallucis longus, and extensor digitorum longus tendons (Fig. 4–10, see also Chapter 3). The dorsalis pedis artery and lesions of the deep peroneal nerve may also be investigated.

Because sonography is a dynamic examination, the foot can be everted, inverted, dorsiflexed, and plantar-flexed during the examination, thus helping to extend the tendon in question and visualize it better, as well as to evoke possible tendon subluxation and episodic impingement (1) (Fig. 4-1).

The tendons should be examined to assess their position and morphology. The normal relationships of the medial, lateral, and anterior compartment tendons vary according to the anatomic positions. Tendons about the ankle are best evaluated in short axis. Subtle areas of tendinosis, cystic degeneration, longitudinal splits, and tendon sheath effusions are best appreciated in this image plane (2) (Figs. 4-11 to 4–15). Abnormalities should be documented in two planes, if possible, to establish their full extent (Figs. 4-16 to 4–18). Extended field of view imaging can be of value in this regard (Figs. 4-19 to 4-23). Recognition of normal

(Text continues on page 44)

A

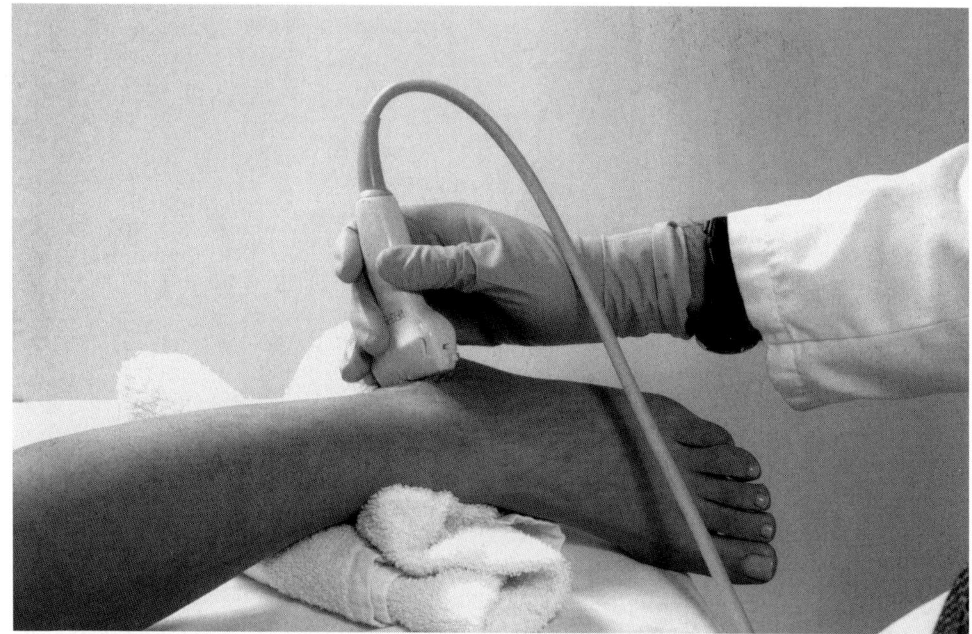

B

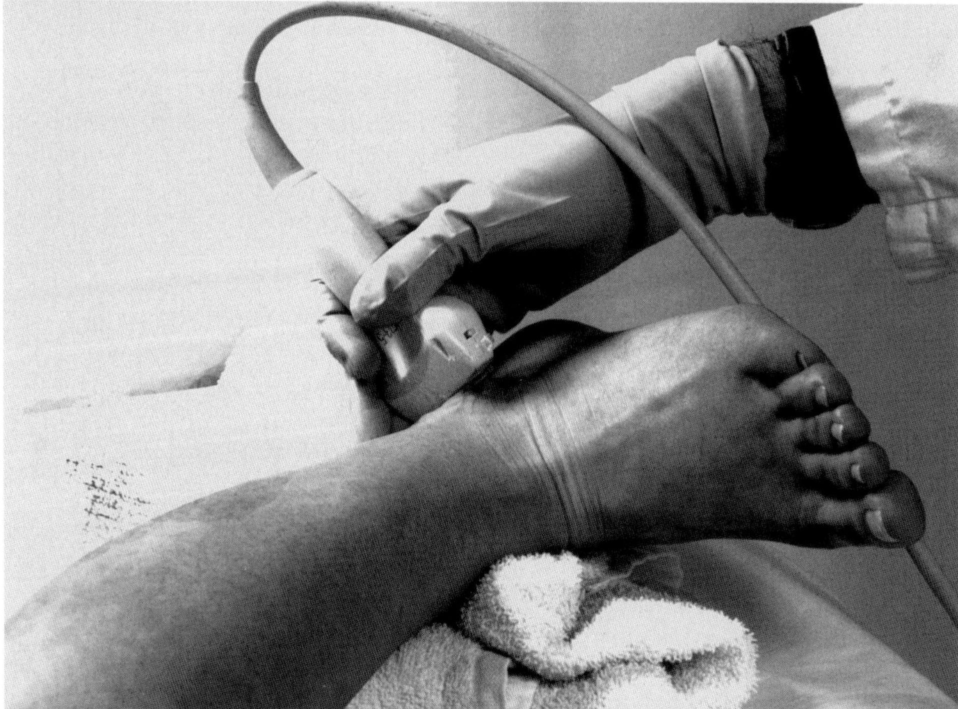

FIG. 4-1. A: Proper transducer positioning for obtaining a transverse image of the peroneal tendons. The transducer is positioned posterior to the lateral malleolus in the anatomic axial plane. **B:** One advantage of sonography is its dynamic capabilities. During real time evaluation, peroneal subluxation or impingement can be evaluated. While keeping the transducer on the lateral aspect of the ankle and having the patient actively evert and dorsiflex the foot, one can observe peroneal subluxation during real time. Subluxation is best assessed while examining the tendons in short axis.

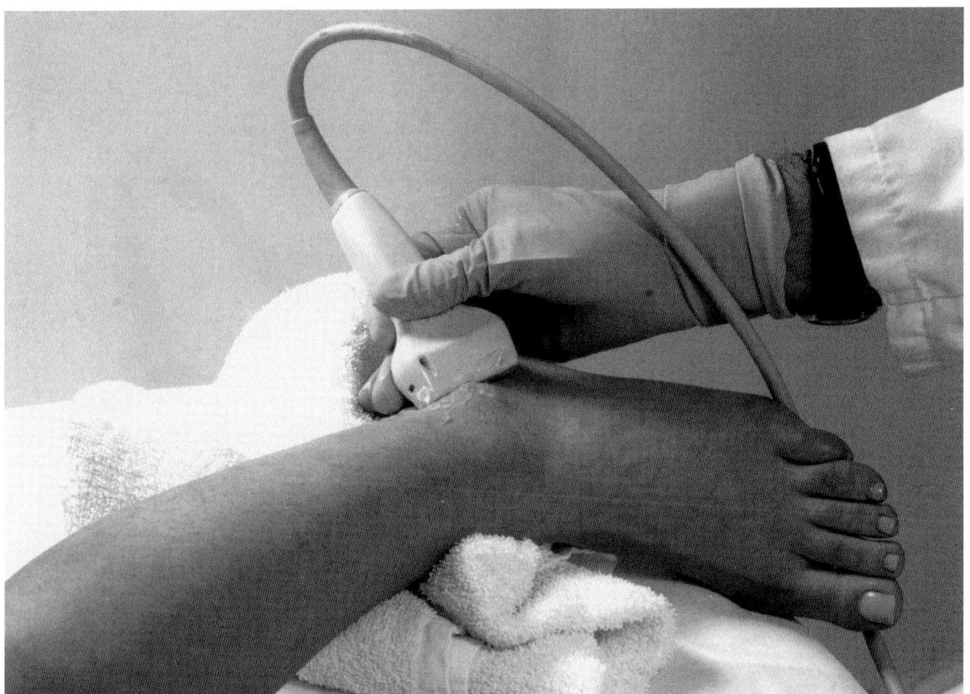

C

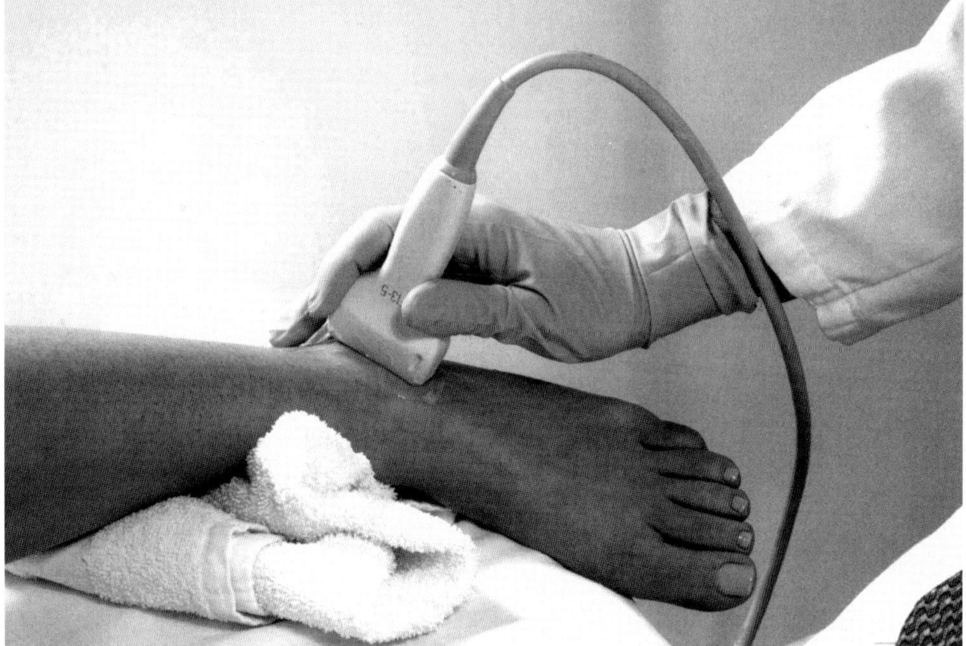

D

FIG. 4-1. C: Care should be taken to align the transducer appropriately along the course of the peroneal tendons, which often involves angling the transducer deep to the lateral malleolus to avoid anisotropy. **D:** Sliding the transducers anteriorly over the fibular enables examination of the anterolateral stabilizers, including the anterior tibiofibular and talofibular ligaments.

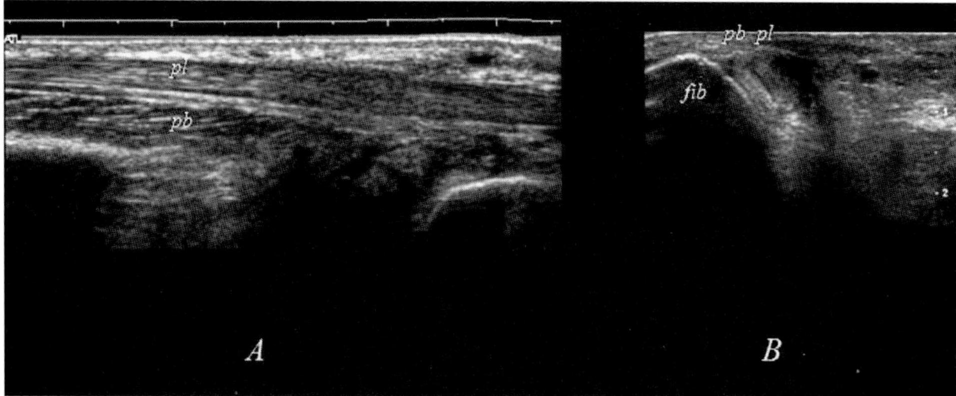

FIG. 4-2. A: Normal longitudinal appearance of the peroneal tendons. Note the normally uniform, hyperechoic bands of tissue with linear internal fibrillar architecture. The peroneus longus (PL) is typically lateral and superficial to the peroneus brevis (PB) at the level of the fibula. In this extended field of view image, a portion of the peroneus brevis muscle is depicted. **B:** Transverse ultrasound image at the tip of the fibula demonstrates the normal appearance of the peroneus longus (PL) as well as the peroneus brevis (PB) tendons, seen in cross section. Note the normal relationship of the peroneal tendons to the fibular groove (fib).

bony landmarks is important, as are normal variants (Fig. 4-24). Impingement or subluxations by indwelling orthopedic hardware should be assessed (Figs. 4-25 and 4-26). Sonography can help elucidate causes of ankle pain in confusing clinical scenarios such as nonspecific focal swelling, which can be caused by tendinosis, an ankle sprain, tibiotalar effusion, or tenosynovitis or cellulitis (Figs. 4-27 and 4-28). Moreover, in cases of suspected infection, ultrasound can help define the presence of an ankle joint effusion as well as guide arthrocentesis and identify other sources of infection such as localized tenosynovitis. This becomes important when septic arthritis is suspected clinically and fluoroscopically guided arthrocentesis is performed; one may pass a needle through a potentially infected tendon sheath and infect an aseptic joint.

The major ligamentous stabilizers about the ankle can be identified with sonography (3) (Figs. 4-3 and 4-7). Most commonly involved in cases of ankle sprains is the anterior talofibular ligament (ATF) (Figs. 4-29 and 4-30). The ATF is best visualized with a high-frequency linear transducer, with the foot inverted and slightly plantar flexed (Fig. 4-1). The probe is held in an oblique coronal projection just inferior to the fibular tip, anteriorly. The anterior talofibular ligament is normally seen as a compact hyperechoic band of tissue with a small amount of surrounding fat (Fig. 4-3). Ligamentous sprains may give rise to a thickened amorphous ligament with an adjacent lateral gutter effusion (Fig. 4-28). Complete acute tears of the ATF are identified as complete ligamentous discontinuity, often with a moderate amount of effusion in the lateral gutter. More chronic remodeled ATFs are thickened and slightly more hypoechoic than normal. In the setting of an inversion injury, avulsion fractures of the involved bony structures should be sought as part of the routine examination (Fig. 4-31). The calcaneofibular ligament (CFL) forms an inferior and medial sling in the inframalleolar region (Fig. 4-3). The transducer is positioned in the posterior oblique coronal plane, visualizing the peroneal tendons in cross section. The ligament is situated medial to the two tendons.

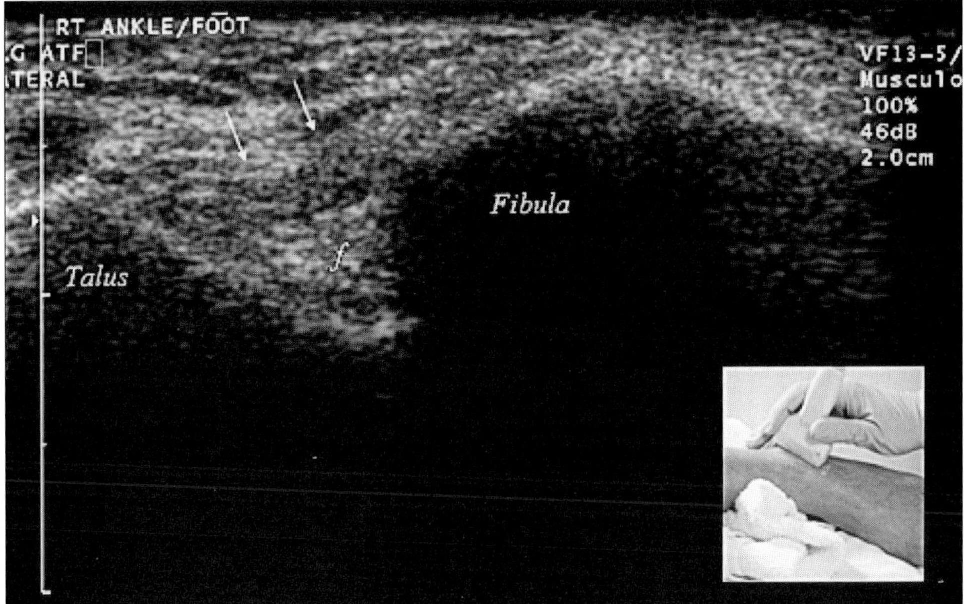

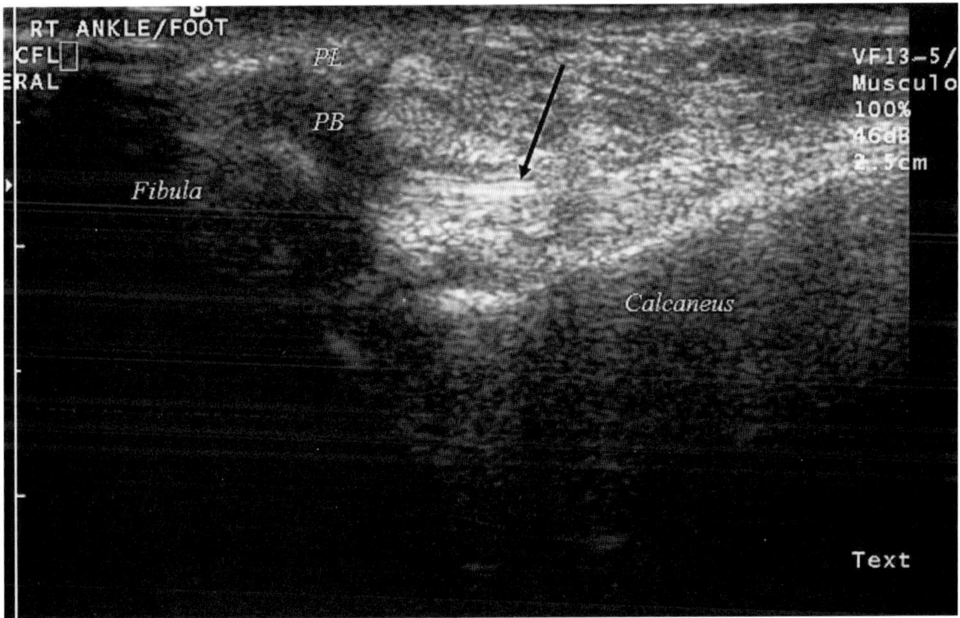

FIG. 4-3. A: The normal anterior talofibular ligament (*arrows*) appears as a thin echogenic band of tissue, which may be difficult to separate from the fat (f) in the lateral gutter on ultrasound. The fibula and talus are labeled. **B:** Transverse view of the lateral ankle demonstrates the normal relationship between the peroneal tendons (PB and PL) and the calcaneofibular ligament deep to the tendons (*arrow*). The calcaneus and fibula are indicated for reference.

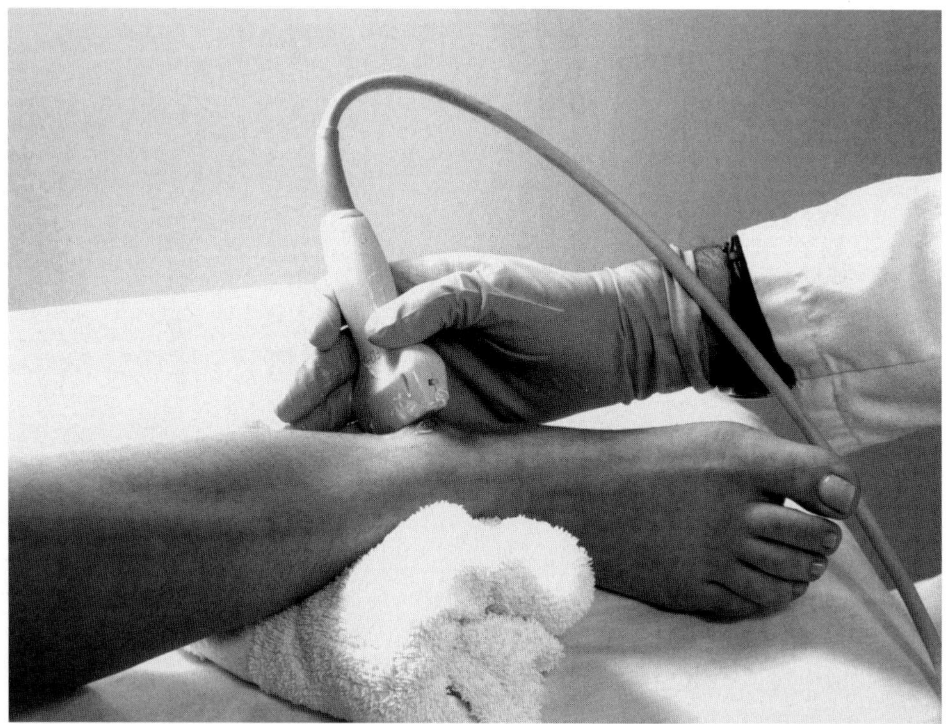

A

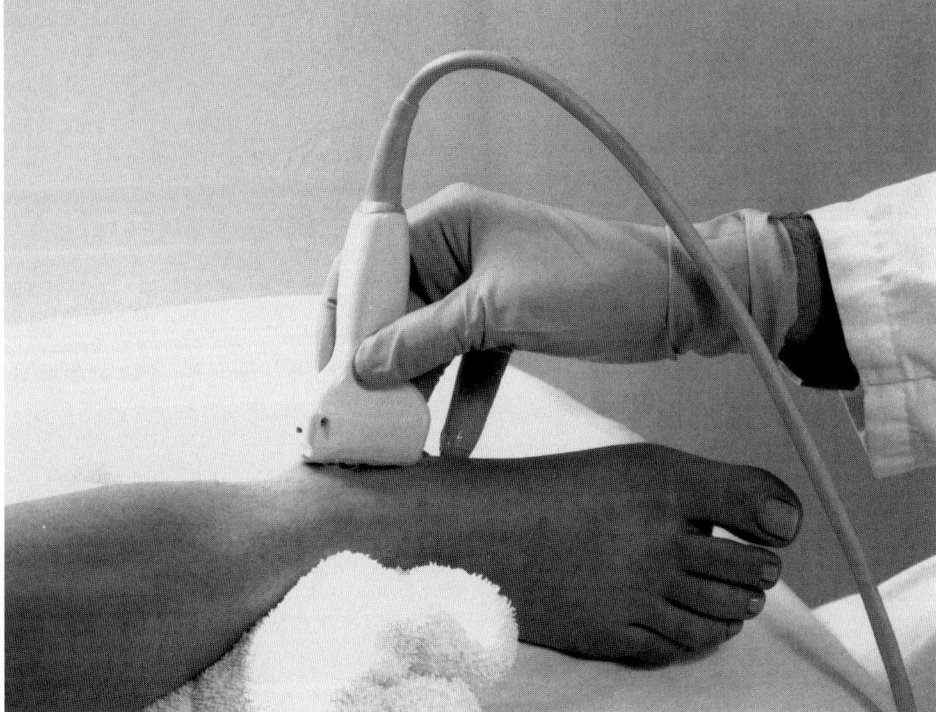

B

FIG. 4-4. Proper transducer positioning for imaging the medial (flexor) compartment tendons in short **(A)** and long **(B)** axis. Bolstering the lateral surface of the ankle, placing it in mild eversion, helps elevate the medial aspect of the ankle and provides a more uniform horizontal imaging surface.

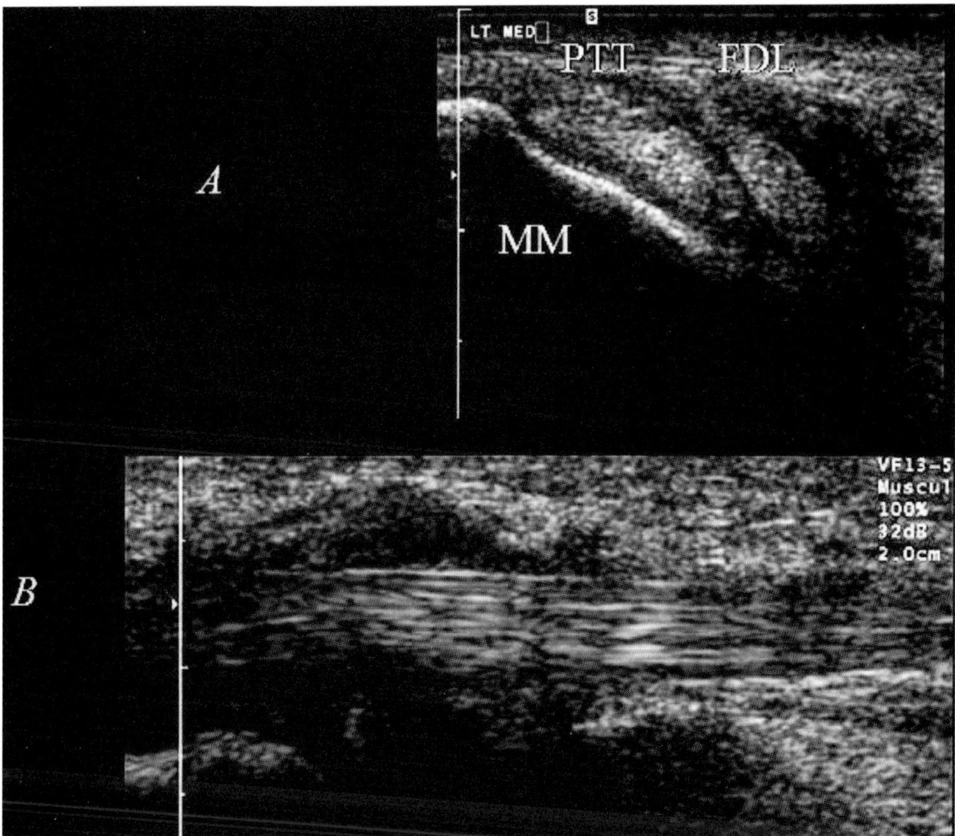

FIG. 4-5. Normal transverse **(A)** and longitudinal **(B)** ultrasound images of the medial aspect of the ankle. The posterior tibial tendon (PTT), as seen in cross section, is typically larger than the flexor digitorum longus (FDL) and flexor hallucis longus tendons. The posterior tibial tendon is anterior to the flexor digitorum longus, and the neurovascular bundle is located posterior to flexor digitorum longus. In **B**, the posterior tibial tendon is shown behind the medial malleolus in long axis.

The deltoid ligament can similarly be examined. The ligament consists of both deep broad fibers (tibiotalar) and a thin superficial component (tibiocalcaneal and tibionavicular fibers) (Fig. 4-6). Loss or normal morphology or discrete defects are indicative of tears (Fig. 4-32).

Normally, minimal, if any, fluid is seen in the tibiotalar joint, generally measuring less than 3 mm as visualized from an anterior approach (4) (Fig. 4-33). Even a small tibiotalar joint effusion can be identified with sonography (5). A medium- or higher-frequency linear probe can be employed, and the approach to the tibiotalar joint is usually from an anterior parasagittal approach, avoiding the dorsalis pedis artery, or from a short axis (lateral or medial) approach (Fig. 4-34).

(Text continues on page 72)

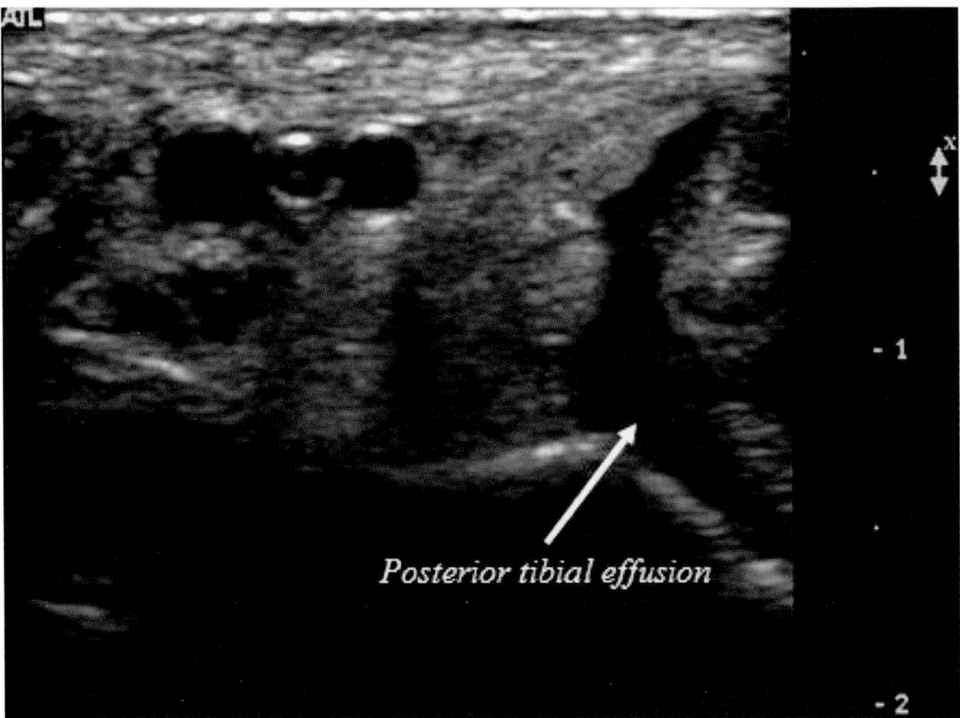

FIG. 4-6. In this transverse image (anatomic axial plane) obtained over the medial compartment, the posterior tibial tendon and flexor digitorum longus tendons (**right**) are separated by fluid in their common tendon sheath (*arrow*). The neurovascular bundle can be seen to the **left** of the image. Three rounded hypoechoic structures correspond to the centrally positioned posterior tibial arteries and adjacent veins. An elliptical hypoechoic structure posterior to the vascular structures, containing fine internal structure, corresponds to the posterior tibial nerve. The surrounding echogenic halo corresponds to the investing fibroadipose connective tissue (or epineurium). The degree to which the nerve appears hypoechoic is variable.

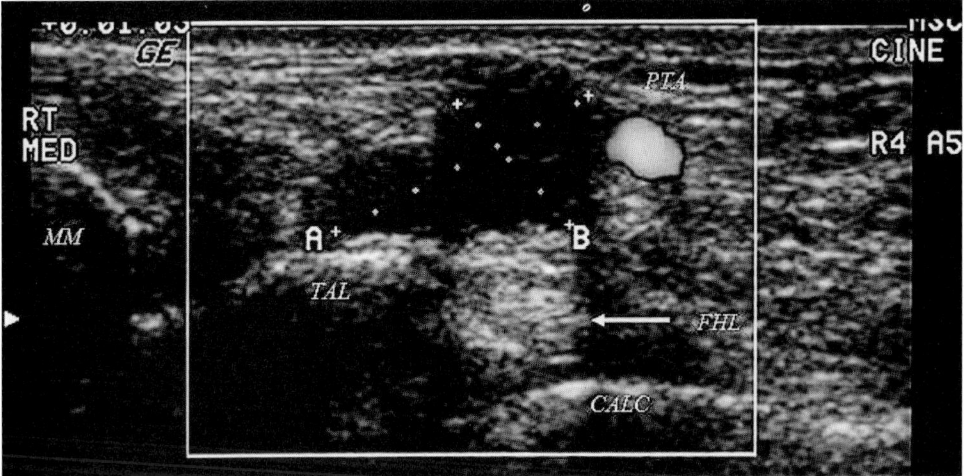

FIG. 4-7. Coronal ultrasound image over the medial compartment in a patient with forefoot paresthesias. A bilobed cystic mass is present (measured) in the expected location of the neurovascular bundle, giving rise to compression of the posterior tibial nerve. The medial malleolus (MM), talus (TAL), calcaneus (CALC), and flexor hallucis longus (FHL) are labeled. Flow is present in the posterior tibial artery (PTA) on power Doppler (shown in *gray scale*).

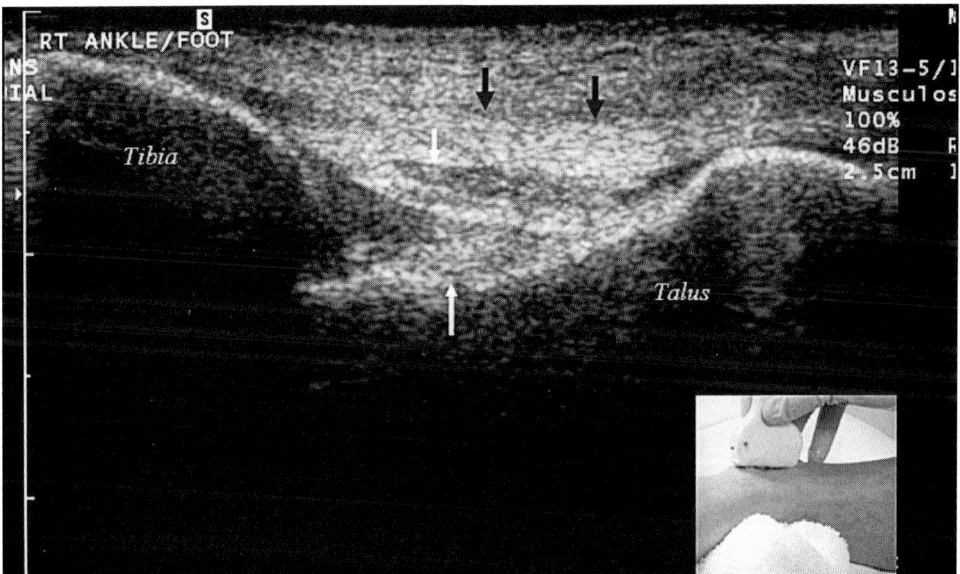

FIG. 4-8. Normal sonographic appearance of the deltoid ligament. The deltoid ligament is normally seen as a compact triangular hyperechoic band of tissue, in continuity between the medial malleolus and the talus (deep fibers, *short white arrows*) and a superficial component (*black arrows*) extending to the calcaneus and navicular bone. These separate components may be difficult to distinguish.

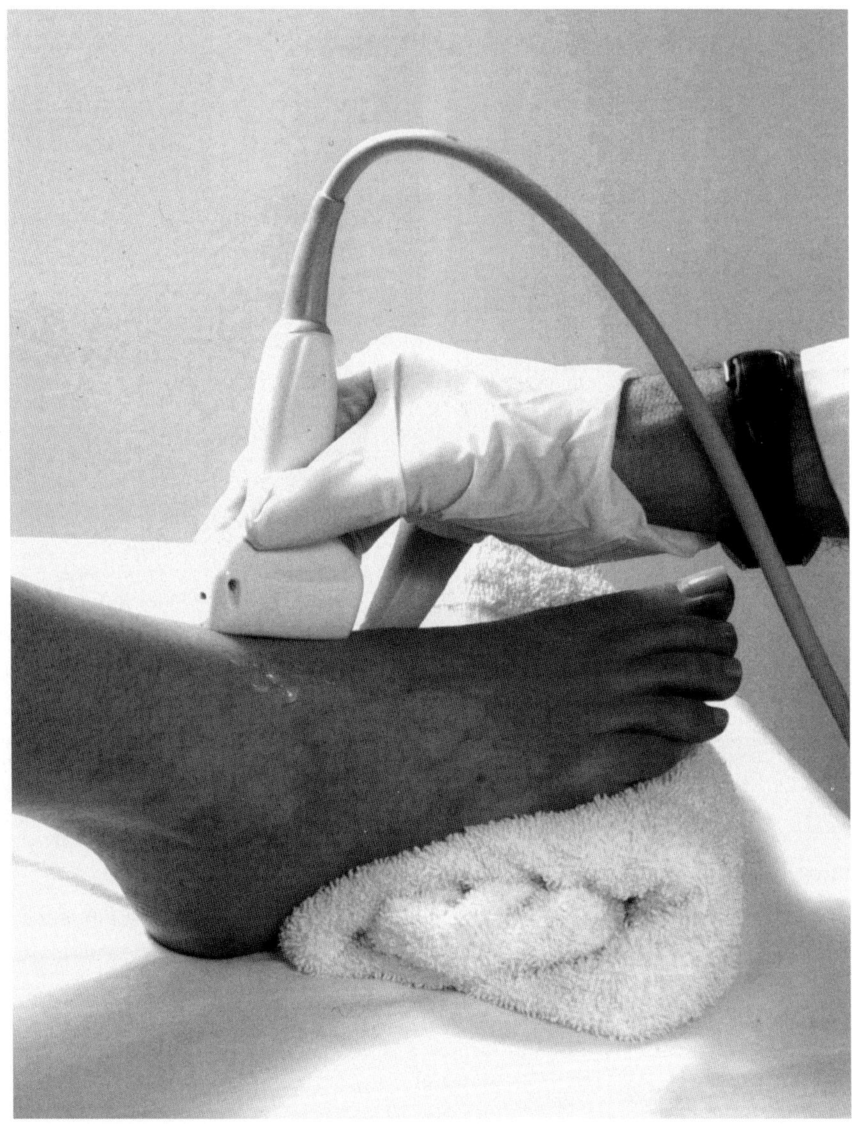

A

FIG. 4-9. A: Proper transducer positioning for obtaining a longitudinal image of the anterior compartment structures. Sweeping the transducer from medial to lateral will allow investigation of the extensor tendons in long axis as well as the dorsalis pedis, deep peroneal nerve, and tibiotalar joint.

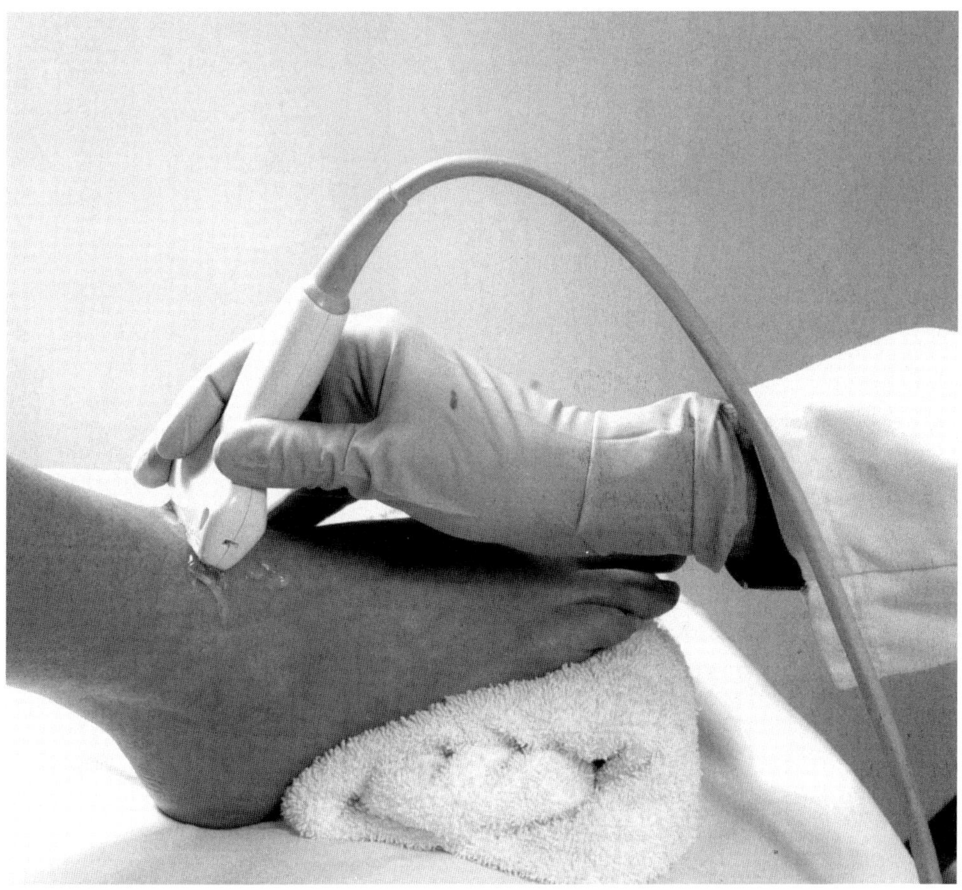

B

FIG. 4-9. B: Proper transducer positioning to obtain a transverse image of the anterior compartment structures.

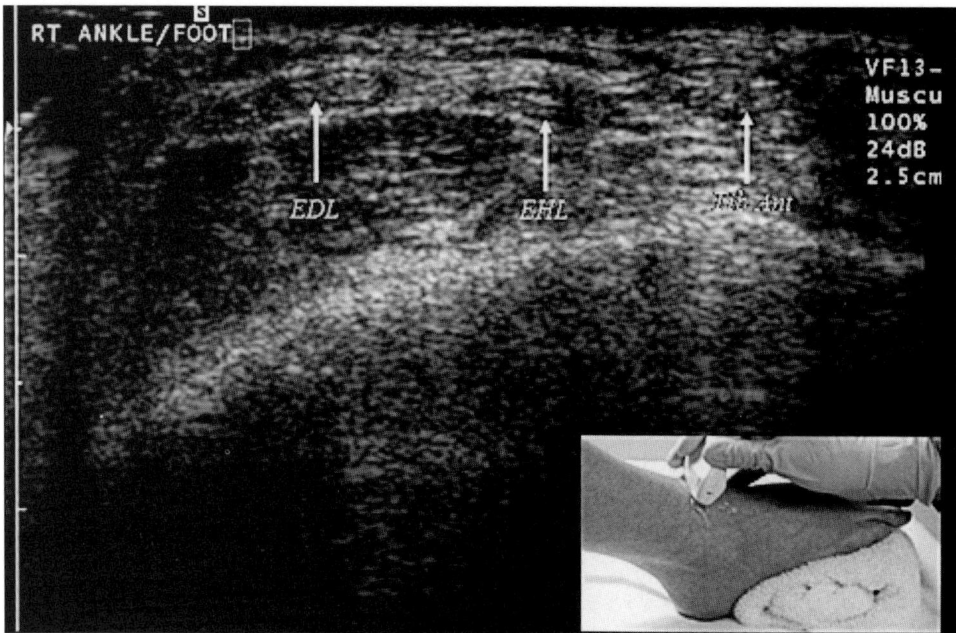

FIG. 4-10. Normal sonographic appearance of the anterior compartment tendons at the level of the anterior compartment. The tibialis anterior (Tib Ant), extensor hallucis longus (EHL), and extensor digitorum longus (EDL) tendons can all be seen in cross section as elliptical echogenic structures.

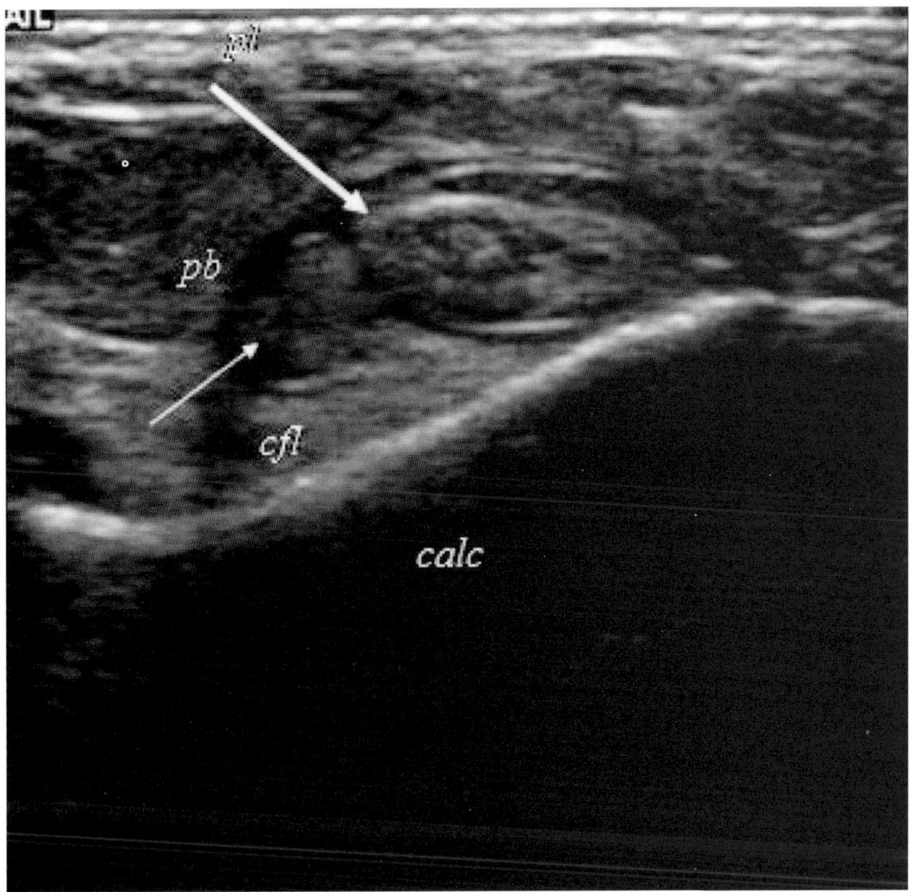

FIG. 4-11. Subtle areas of tendinosis are best appreciated in short axis as illustrated in this image of the peroneal tendons (labeled), which was obtained at the level of the calcaneofibular ligament (cfl). The peroneus brevis (pb) is mildly inhomogeneous, and the peroneus longus (pl) contains thin intrasubstance hypoechoic clefts. The calcaneus (calc) is indicated.

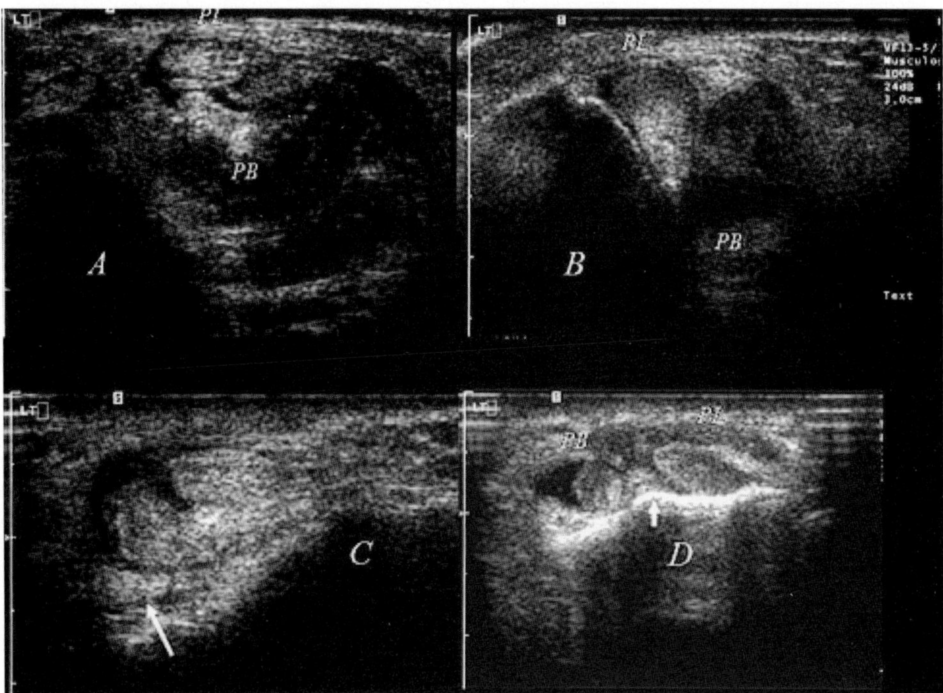

FIG. 4-12. The tendons should be followed using a systematic approach in short axis from origin to insertion. These images represent short axis views of the peroneal tendons, **(A)** above the lateral sulcus, **(B)** at the lateral sulcus, **(C)** at the level of the calcaneofibular ligament, and, **(D)** at the peroneal tubercle (*arrow*) of the calcaneus. At each level, abnormal tendon morphology and tendon sheath fluid or thickening can be appreciated.

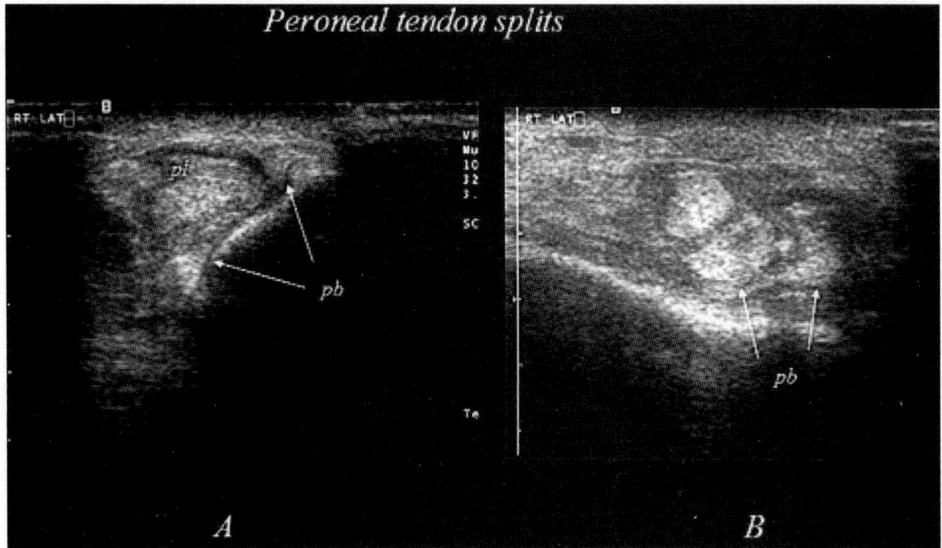

FIG. 4-13. Short axis views of the peroneal tendons at the level of the lateral peroneal sulcus **(A)** and calcaneofibular ligament **(B)**. Both tendons are enlarged, containing longitudinal split tears. There is wide separation of the peroneus brevis fragments (*arrows*) in part **A**, which are in closer apposition distally **(B)**.

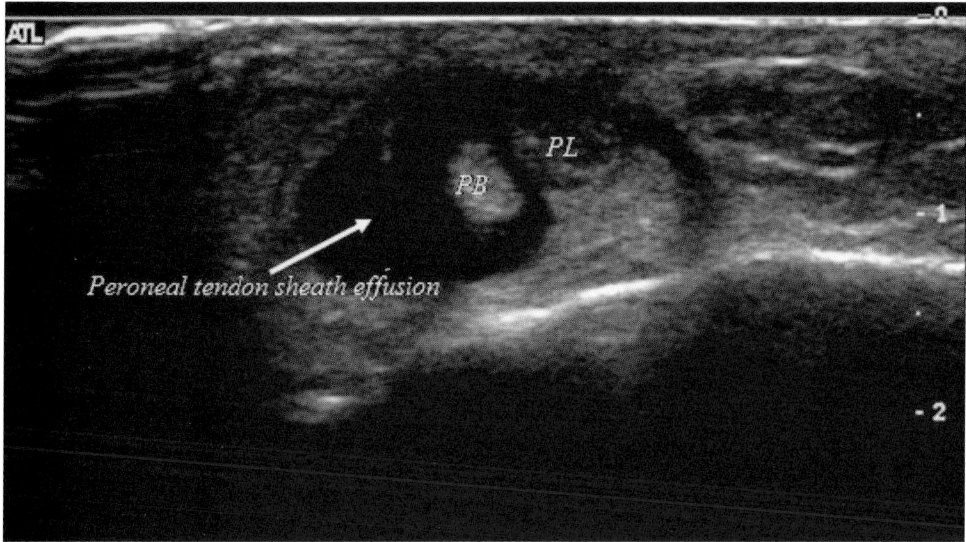

A

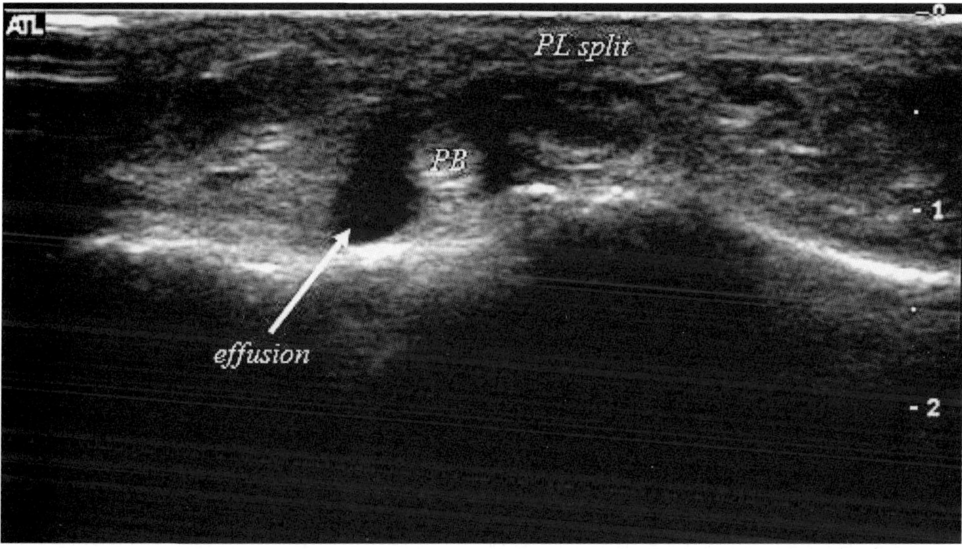

B

FIG. 4-14. A: Short axis ultrasound images along the lateral aspect of the ankle demonstrate tendinosis of the peroneus brevis (PB) and longus (PL) tendons. Moreover, there is a large amount of anechoic fluid surrounding the tendon, consistent with a tendon sheath effusion (effusion). **B:** A slightly more caudal image in the same patient shows a split in the peroneus longus tendon at the level of the peroneal tubercle.

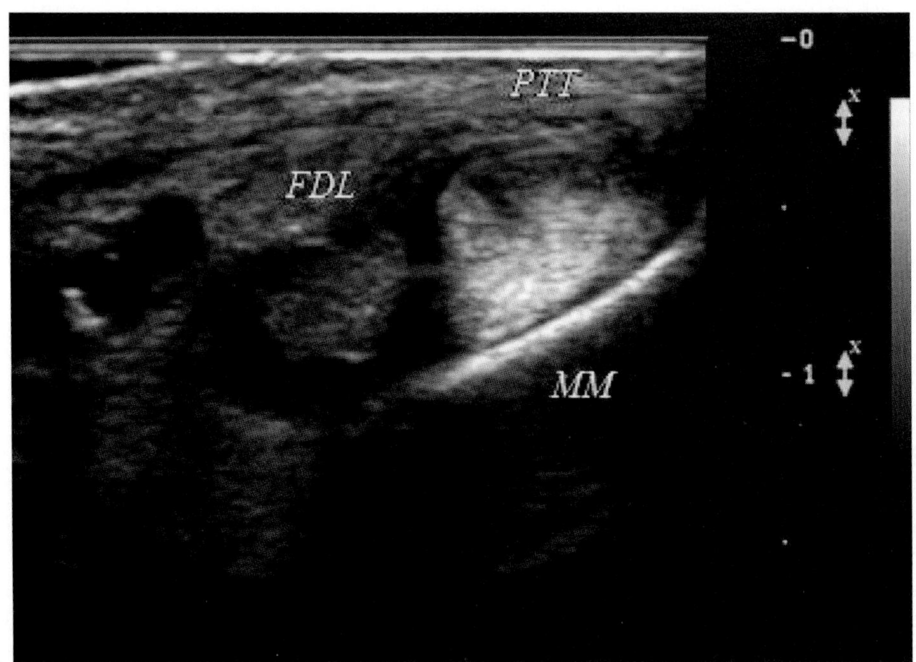

A

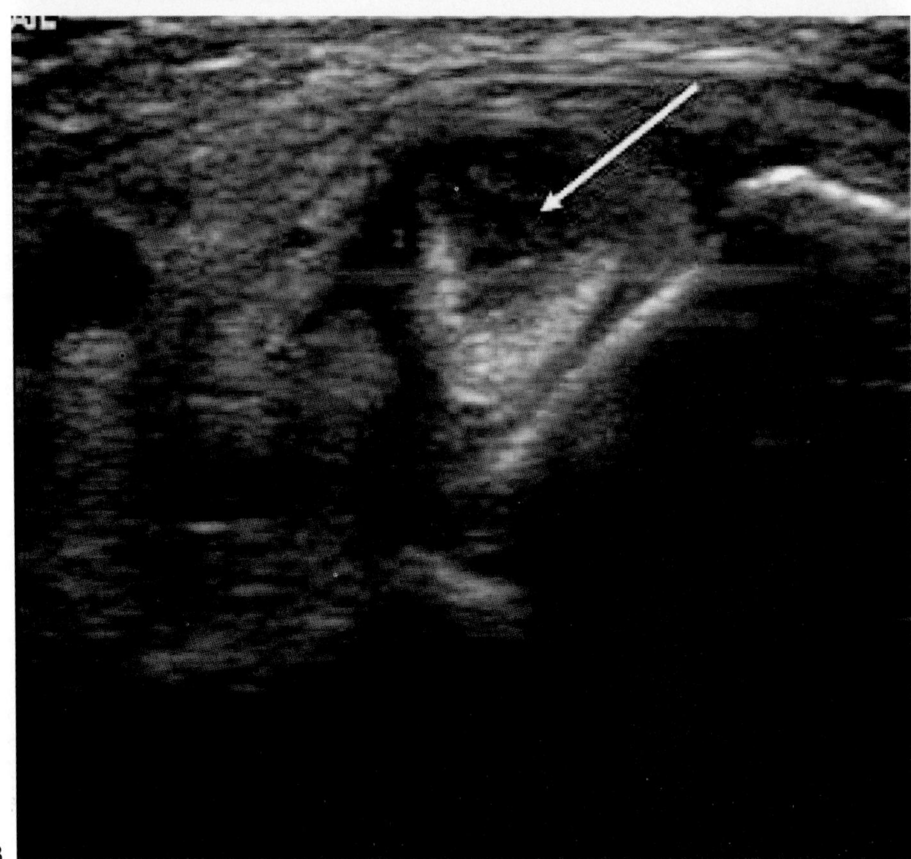

B

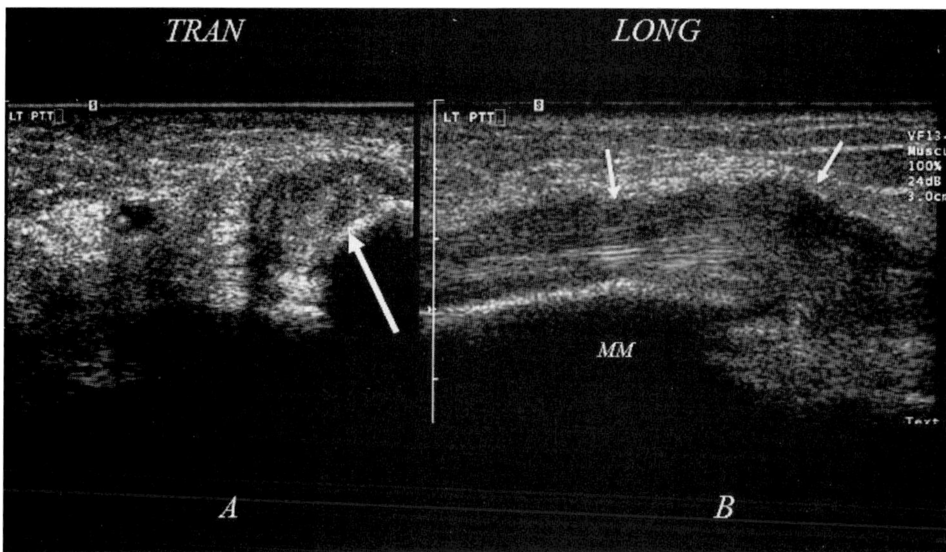

FIG. 4-16. Tendon abnormalities should be imaged in two planes, as indicated in this case of posterior tibial tendinosis. Although short axis views are sensitive to subtle tendinosis, the full extent of the tendinopathy, as well as its relationship to other anatomic landmarks, is better appreciated in long axis. In this case, the short axis view **(A)** shows intrasubstance clefts, enlargement, and indistinct margins of the tendon (*arrow*). In part **B**, one can better appreciate the extent of this abnormality (*arrows*) as the tendon passes over the medial malleolus (MM).

FIG. 4-15. A: Transverse ultrasound image at the tip of the medial malleolus demonstrates tendinosis of the posterior tibial tendon (PTT) and flexor digitorum longus (FDL). The tendons are enlarged, and there is moderate surrounding fluid. Portions of the neurovascular bundle are evident in the **left** of the image. **B:** Transverse ultrasound image of the posterior tibial tendon obtained slightly more caudally in the same patient demonstrates moderate tendinosis of the tendon, with a linear hypoechoic split within the periphery of the tendon (*arrow*).

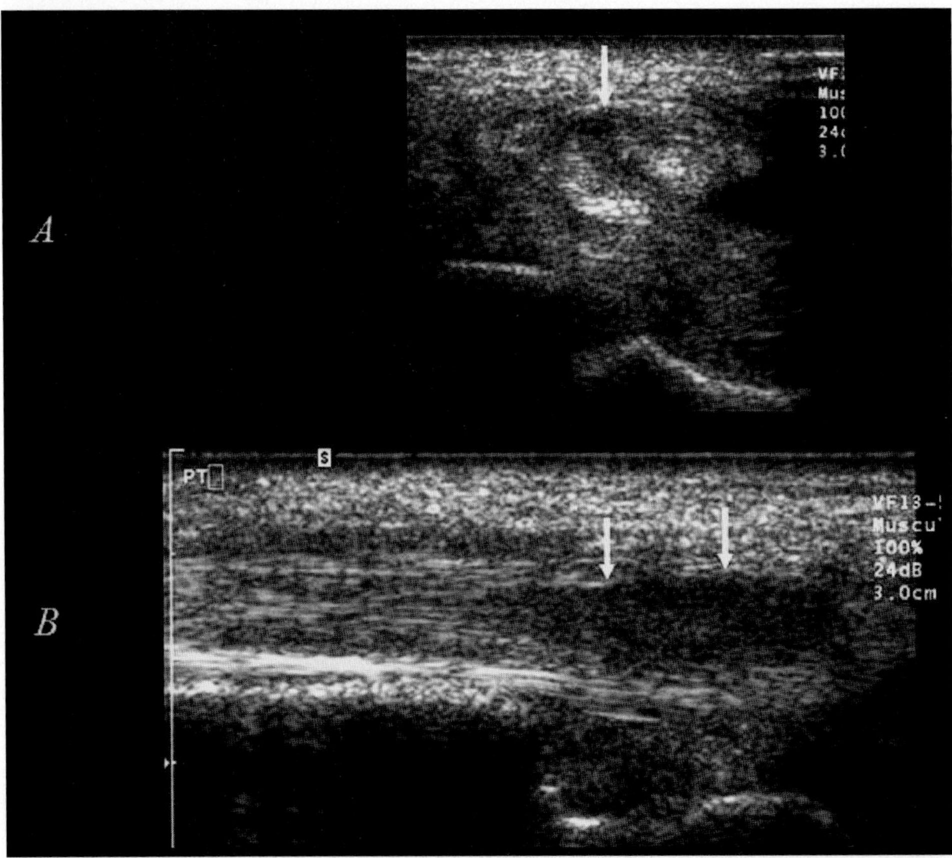

FIG. 4-17. Transverse **(A)** and longitudinal **(B)** images of the posterior tibial tendon showing a full-thickness longitudinal split tear. This appears as an obliquely oriented hypoechoic defect within the tendon substance (*arrows*). The length of the tear is appreciated on the long axis view **(B)**.

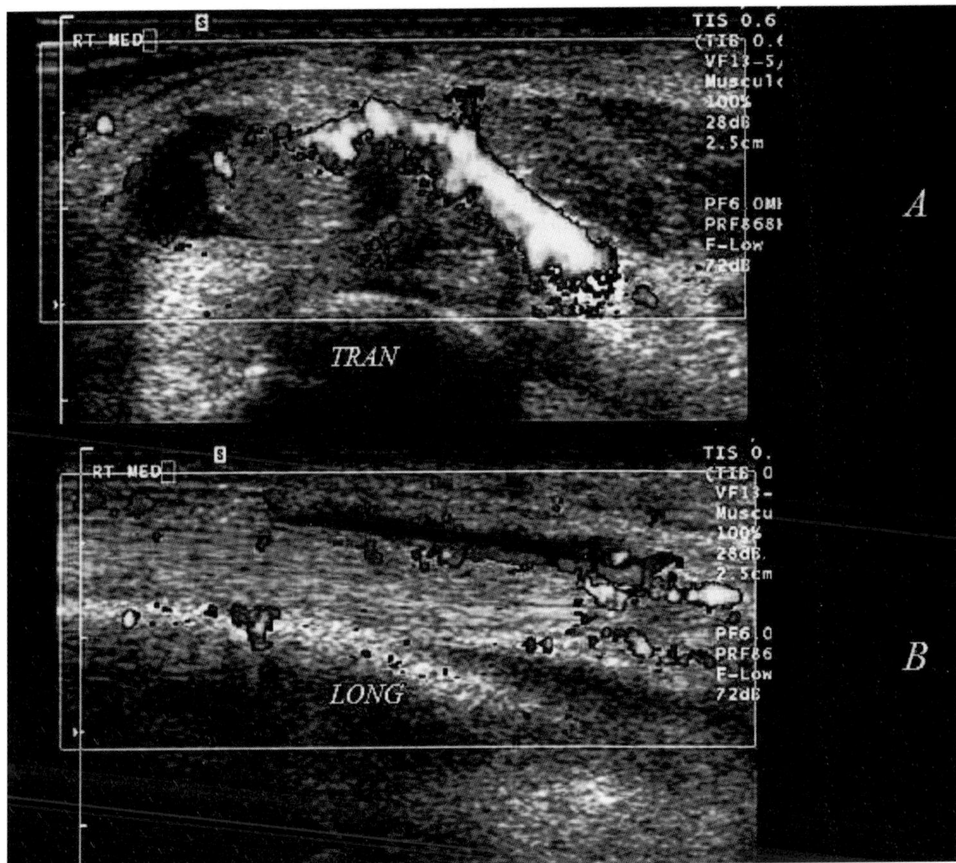

FIG. 4-18. Transverse **(A)** and longitudinal **(B)** ultrasound images of the posterior tibial tendon demonstrating fluid surrounding the tendon, consistent with a tendon sheath effusion. Of note, the application of power Doppler demonstrates increased vascularity, consistent with posterior tibial tenosynovitis.

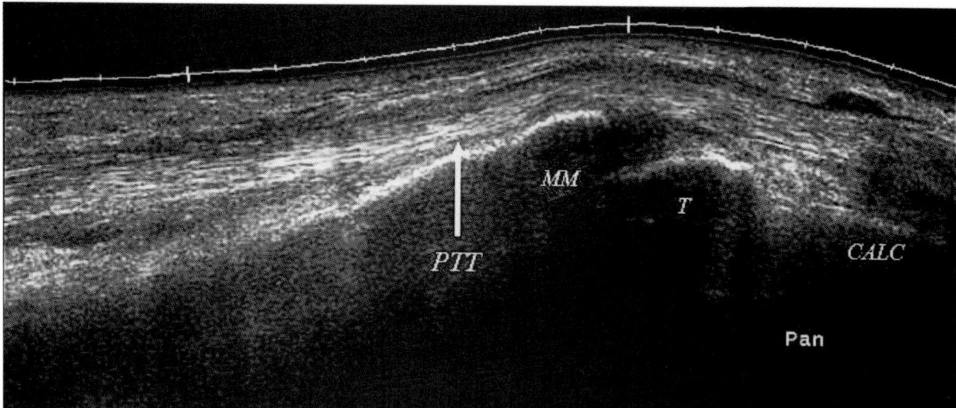

FIG. 4-19. Extended field of view imaging allows depiction of the full extent of abnormality. This longitudinal extended field of view image along the medial aspect of the ankle in a patient with posterior tibial tendinosis (PTT) demonstrates the extent of the abnormal tendon segment, the relationship between the tendon and the adjacent osseous structures: medial malleolus (MM), talus (T), and calcaneus (CALC). Note the focal distention of the distal tendon sheath (**right**).

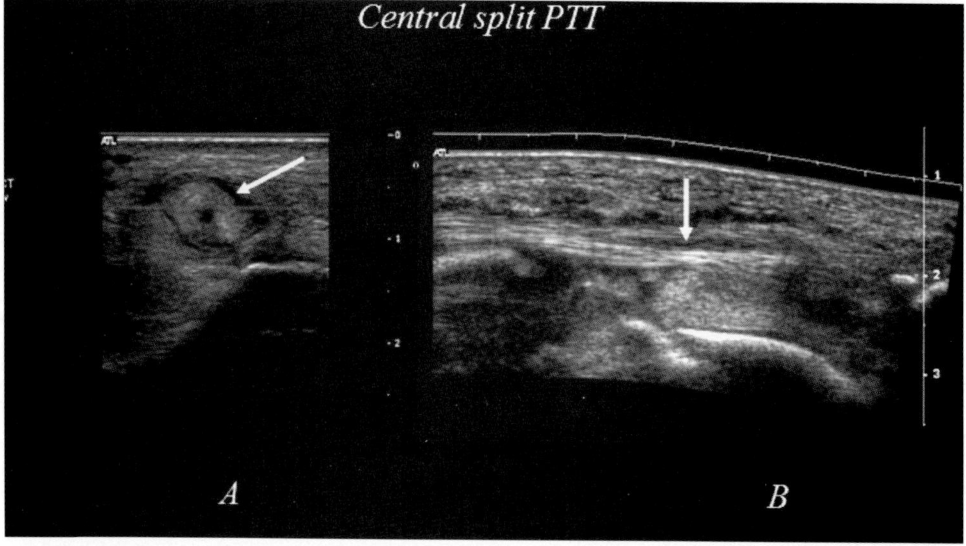

FIG. 4-20. Short axis **(A)** and extended field of view longitudinal **(B)** images of the posterior tibial tendon demonstrating tendinosis with a central split within the substance of the tendon. There is nodular thickening of the tendon sheath over the entire visualized segment of the tendon.

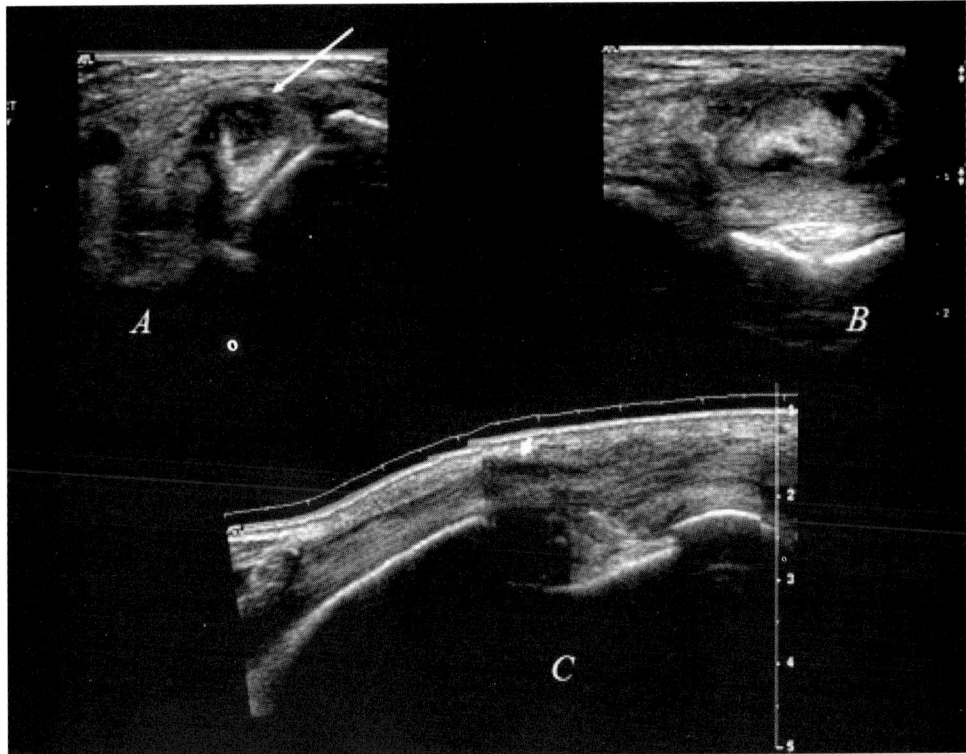

FIG. 4-21. Short axis **(A, B)** and extended field of view long axis **(C)** images of the posterior tibial tendon in a patient with tendinosis and a longitudinal split tear. On short axis, the complex nature of the tears (*arrows*) is appreciated. On extended field of view imaging, the length of the abnormality and location are better depicted. The osseus structures visualized include the medial malleolus and talus.

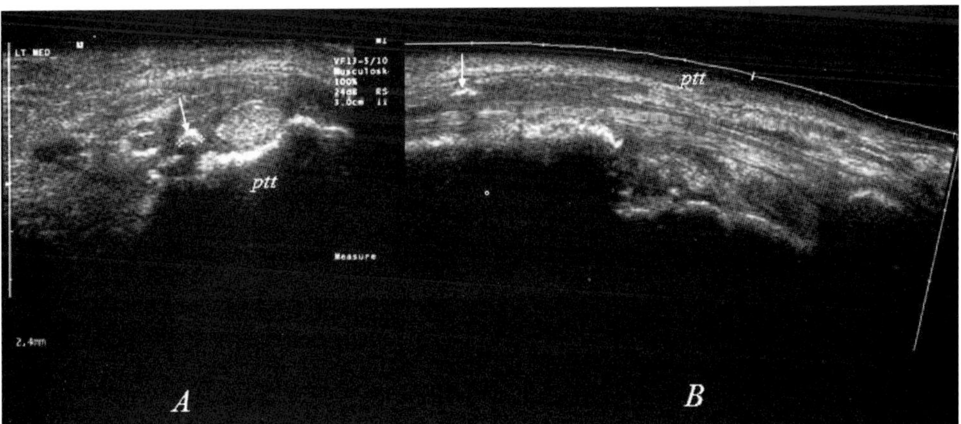

FIG. 4-22. Short axis **(A)** and extended field of view long axis **(B)** images of the posterior tibial tendon (PTT) in a patient with tendinosis and a small osteochondral body (*arrow*). On short axis, there is thickening of the tendon sheath with the small body posterior to the tendon. On extended field of view imaging, the ossific fragment lies above the medial malleolus. The osseus structures visualized include the medial malleolus, talus, and navicular bone. In **B**, the tendon can be traced to its navicular insertion (**right**).

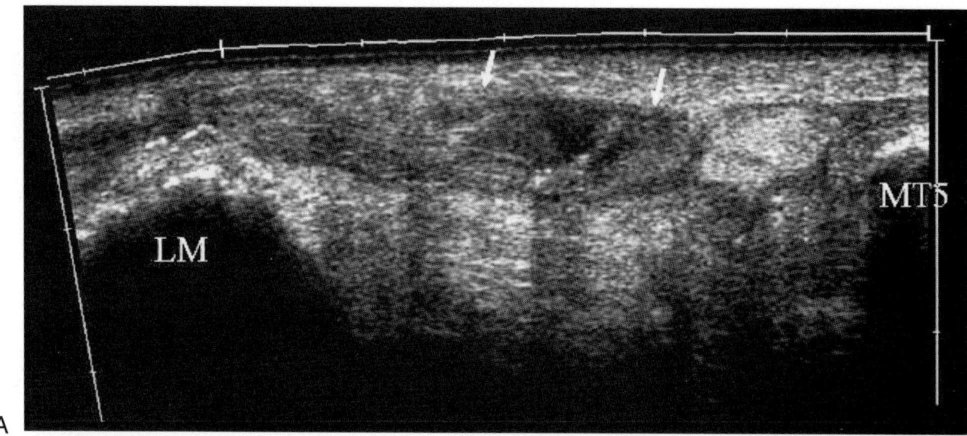

A

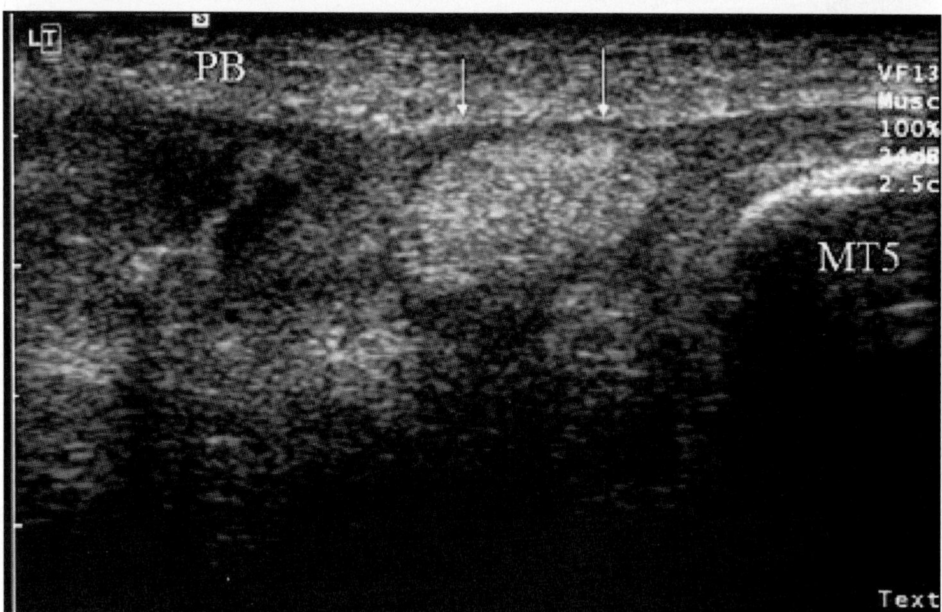

B

FIG. 4-23. A: Longitudinal extended field of view image demonstrates marked distal tendinosis of the peroneus brevis with a high-grade partial tear (*arrows*) just proximal to the insertion at the fifth metatarsal base (MT5). The tendon is retracted and degenerated. The lateral malleolus (LM) is also indicated for reference. **B:** Improved spatial detail is obtained in this longitudinal image demonstrating the same high-grade tear with retraction of the peroneus brevis (*arrows*). The base of the fifth metatarsal (MT5) is indicated.

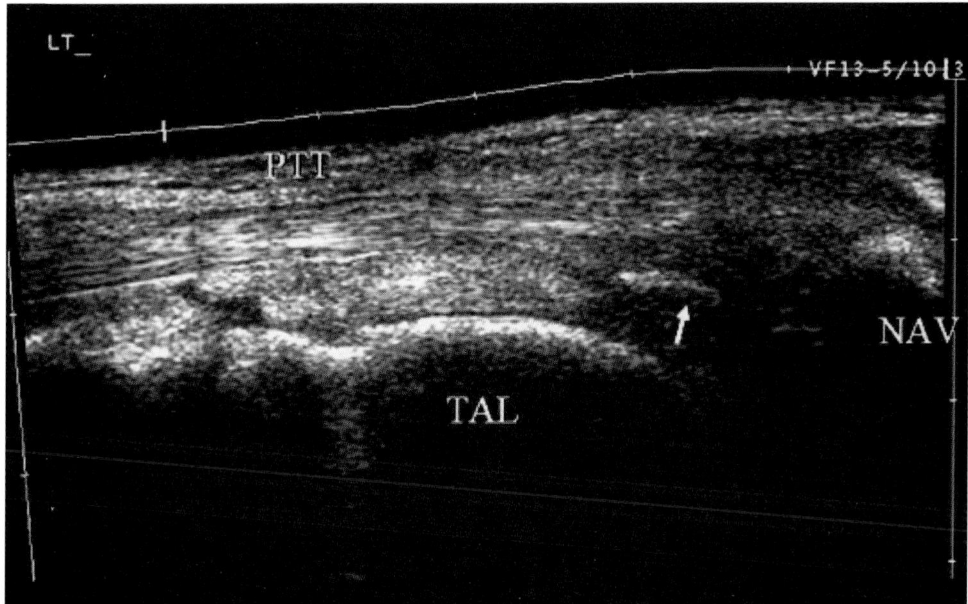

A

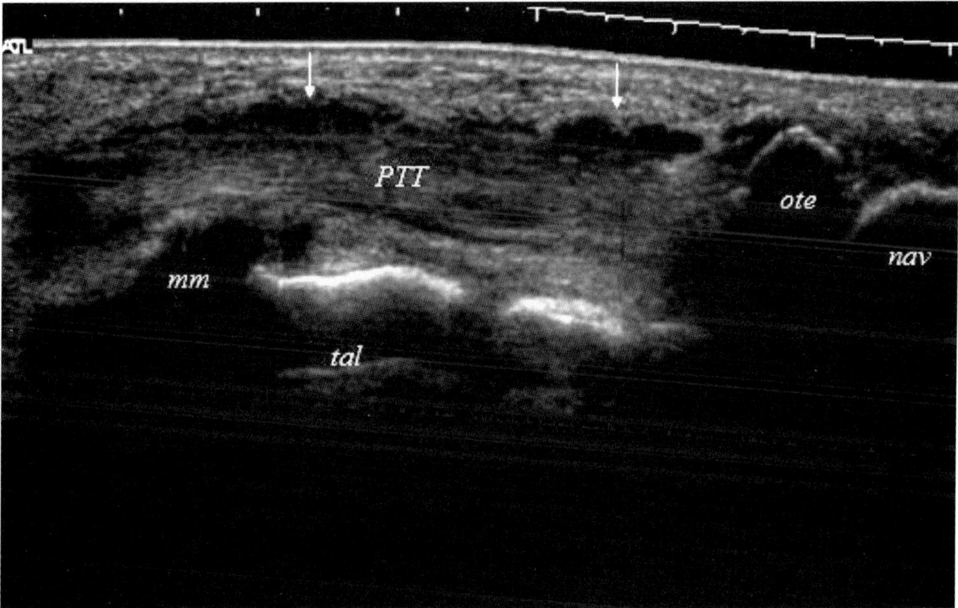

B

FIG. 4-24. Longitudinal extended field of view ultrasound images of the distal posterior tibial tendon (PTT) demonstrate the tendon insertion onto the tarsal navicular. It is not uncommon for an intratendinous ossicle to be present at the insertion site of the posterior tibial tendon. These demonstrate significant variability. It is important to recognize these are normal variants. **A:** A thin ossicle is evident along the deep surface of the tendon (*arrow*) just proximal to its insertion (nav). The talus (tal) is labeled. **B:** A much larger ossicle [os tibiale externum (ote)] is present. Large ossicles may show varying degrees of fibrous or bony union with the adjacent navicular bone (nav), resulting in localized pain. There is moderate degeneration of the distal aspect of the posterior tibial tendon (PTT) with loculated fluid in the tendon sheath (*arrows*).

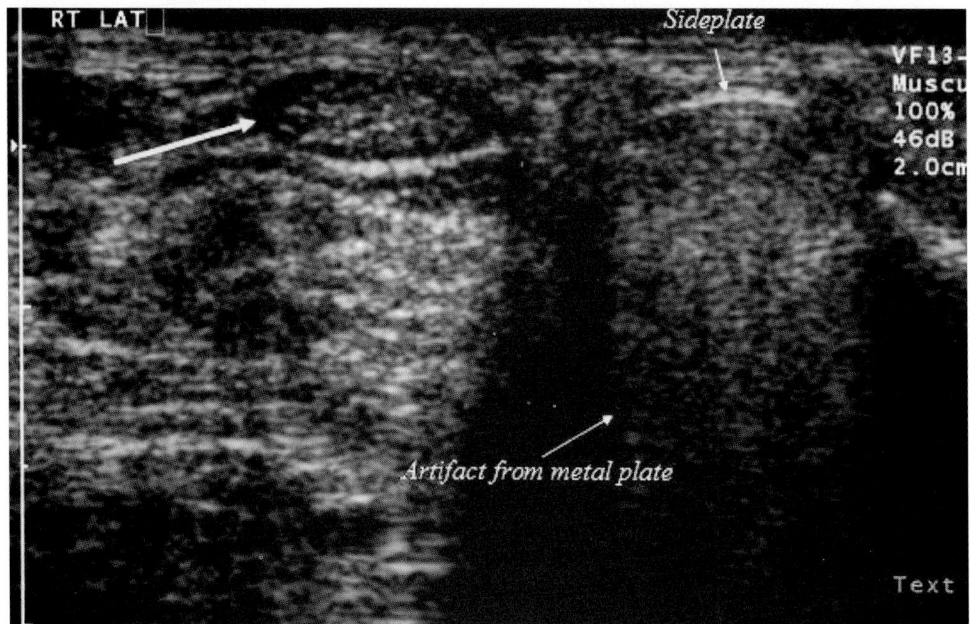

FIG. 4-25. The advantage of sonography in imaging patients with indwelling orthopedic fixation is that evaluation of the soft tissues is not hindered by artifact generated by the hardware. This transverse image along the lateral joint line clearly delineates the peroneus longus (*arrow*) from the adjacent orthopedic side plate. Intervening hypoechoic soft tissue corresponds to a degenerated, hypoechoic peroneus brevis tendon, deformed by the adjacent plate. Note the posterior reverberation artifact from the side plate. The deformity was accentuated with eversion of the ankle.

A

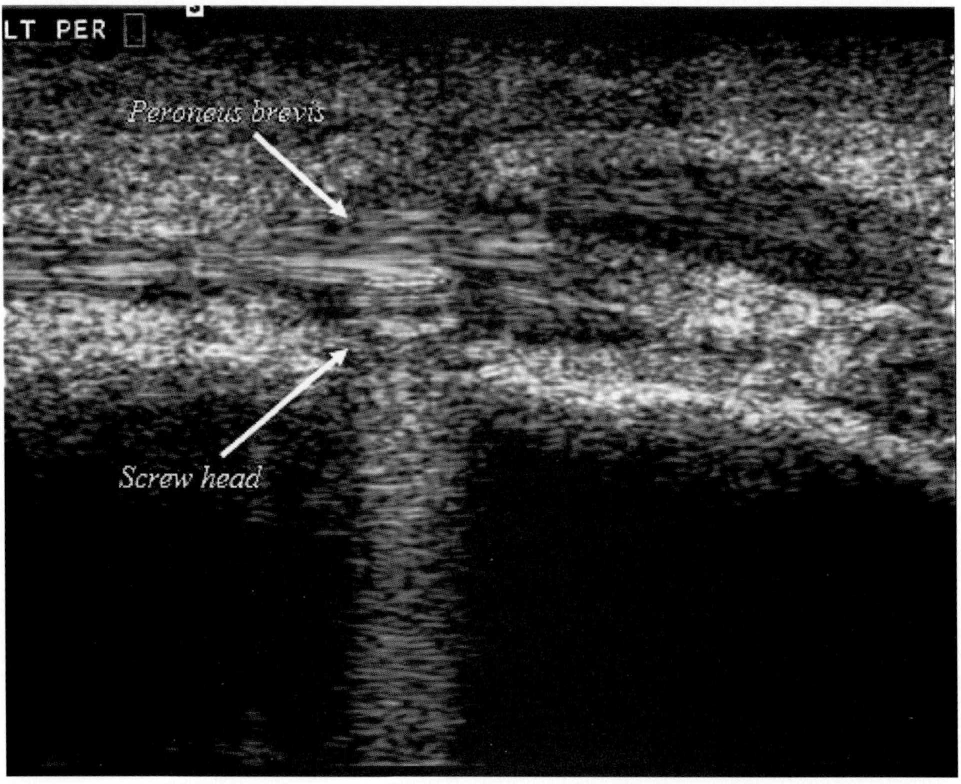

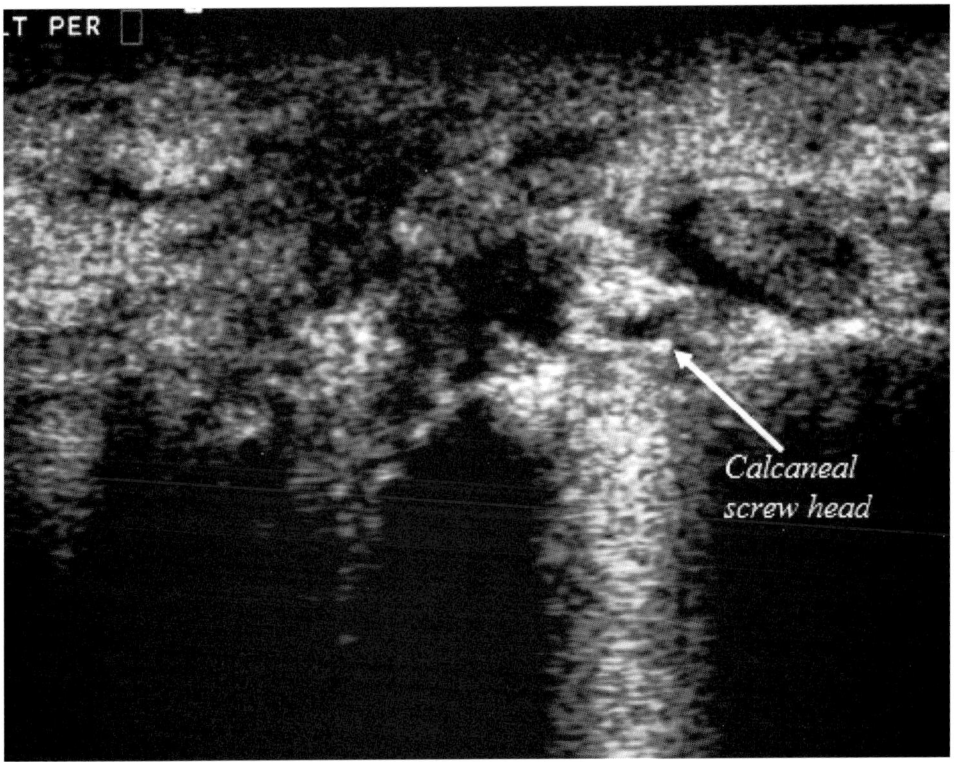

B

FIG. 4-26. B: Transverse image along the lateral joint line in the same patient demonstrates the relationship of the screw head to the deep fibers of the peroneus brevis (*arrow*). The patient described pain localized to the site of screw placement.

FIG. 4-26. A: Longitudinal ultrasound image along the lateral joint line in a patient after internal fixation of a calcaneal fracture with lateral ankle pain. This longitudinal image demonstrates mild tendinosis of the peroneus brevis. Note that the deep fibers of the peroneus brevis are abutting one of the screw heads in the calcaneus.

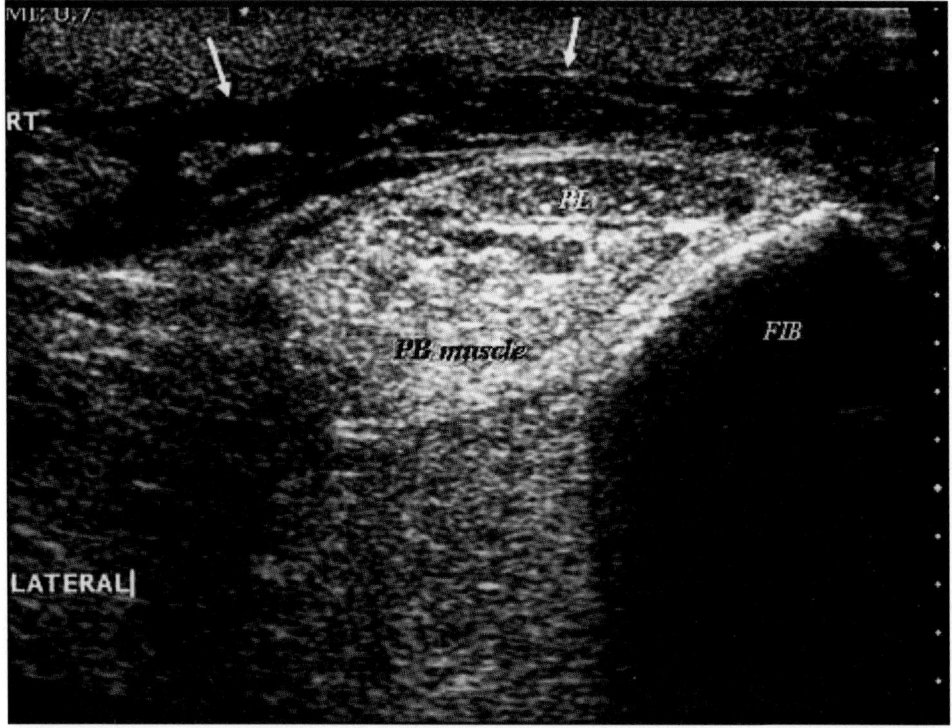

FIG. 4-27. Short axis view obtained along the lateral aspect of the distal leg in a patient with chronic foot drop demonstrates marked atrophy of the peroneus brevis muscle belly (PB muscle), which appears sonographically as loss of muscle bulk and increased echogenicity. The peroneus longus (PL) is labeled. Note the overlying subcutaneous edema (*arrows*) giving rise to the visible soft tissue swelling. No intrinsic tendon abnormality was evident. The fibula (fib) is indicated for reference.

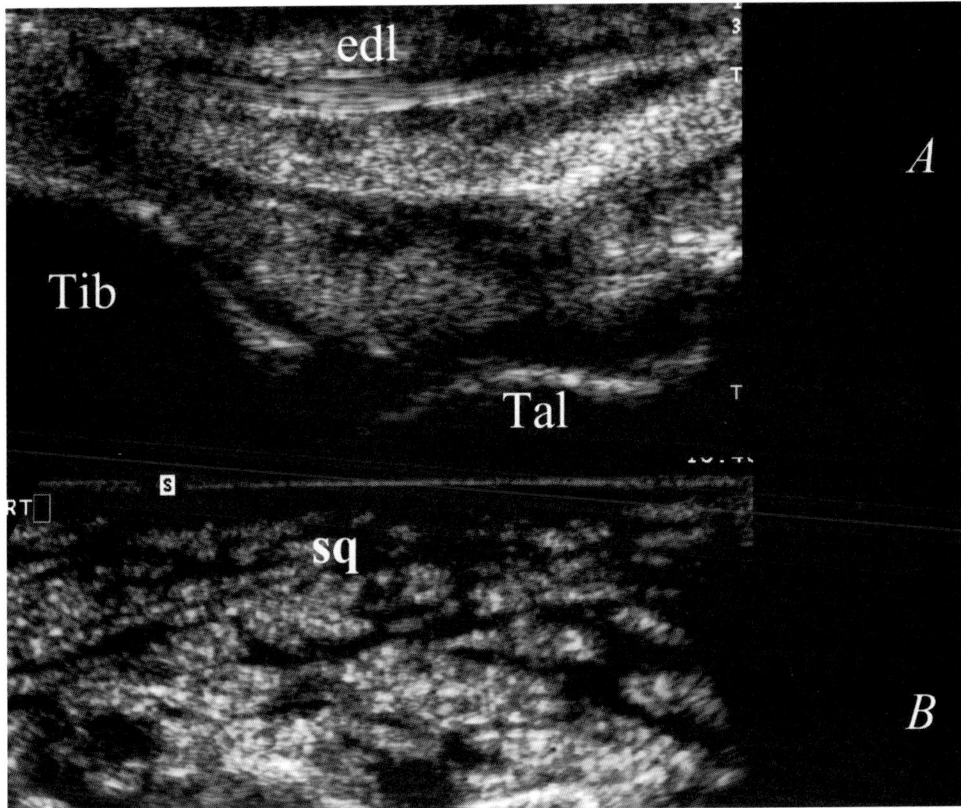

FIG. 4-28. Longitudinal ultrasound images over the dorsal aspect of the ankle show extensive subcutaneous edema. **A:** No significant joint or tendon sheath effusion could be demonstrated. No intrinsic tendon abnormality was present, confirming that swelling was entirely confined to the subcutaneous fat. The extensor digitorum longus (edl), tibia (Tib), and talus (Tal) are labeled. **B:** Extensive serpiginous hypoechoic clefts in the subcutaneous fat are present, representing areas of lymphatic resorption. The surround fat is diffusely echogenic compatible with edema. The patient was subsequently treated for cellulitis.

A

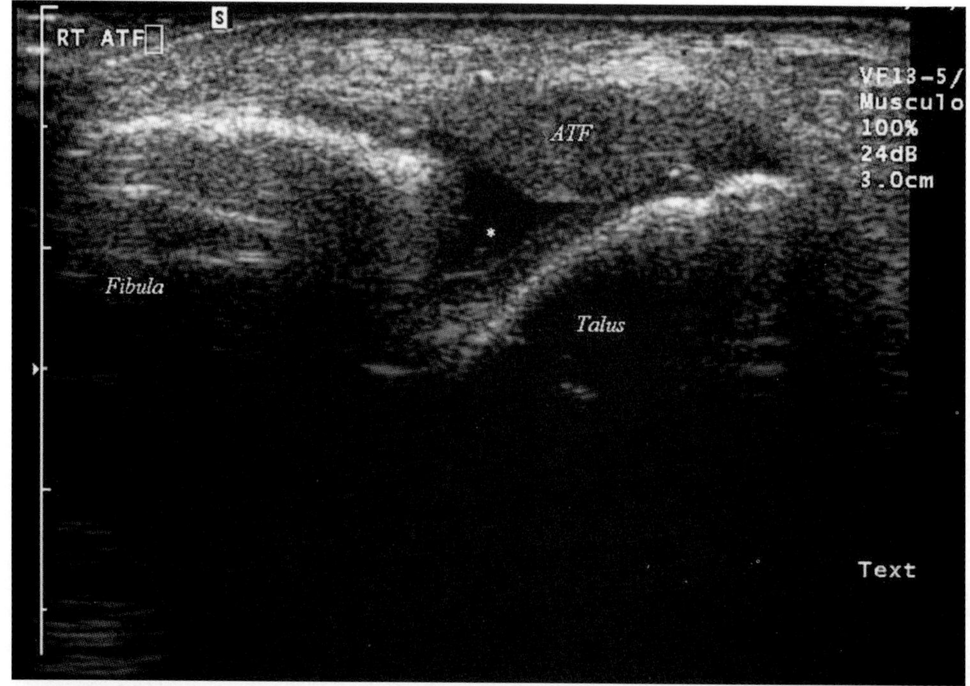

B

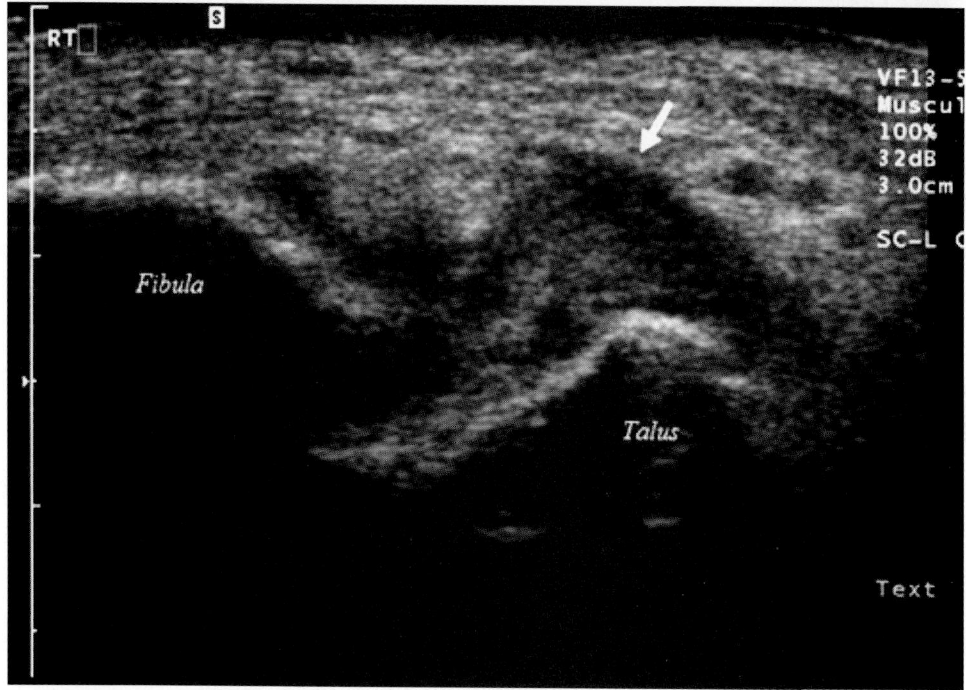

FIG. 4-29. A: Ultrasound image demonstrates marked thickening and decreased echogenicity of the anterior talofibular ligament (ATF), consistent with high-grade partial sprain. Note also the anechoic fluid replacing the normally hyperechoic fat deep to the ligament (*asterisk*). **B:** High-grade partial tear in another patient with history of inversion injury. The fibula and talus are labeled.

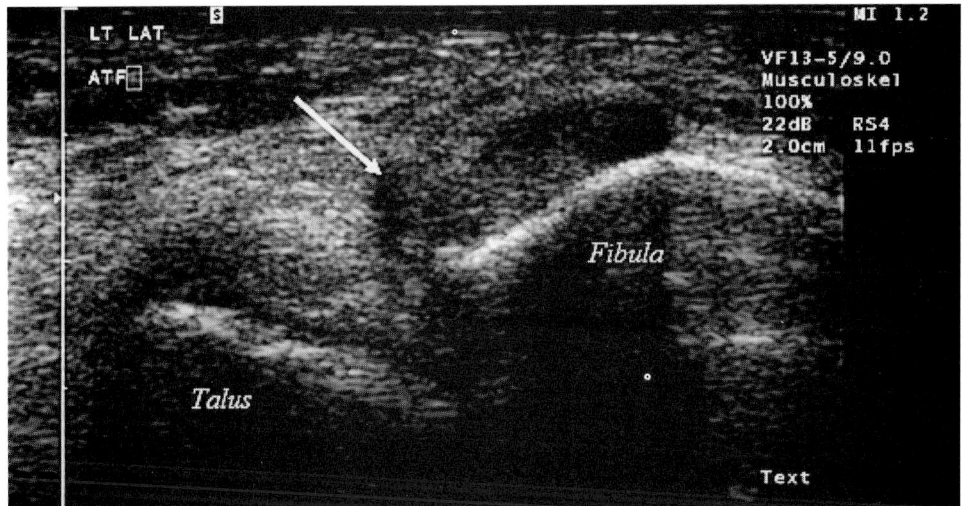

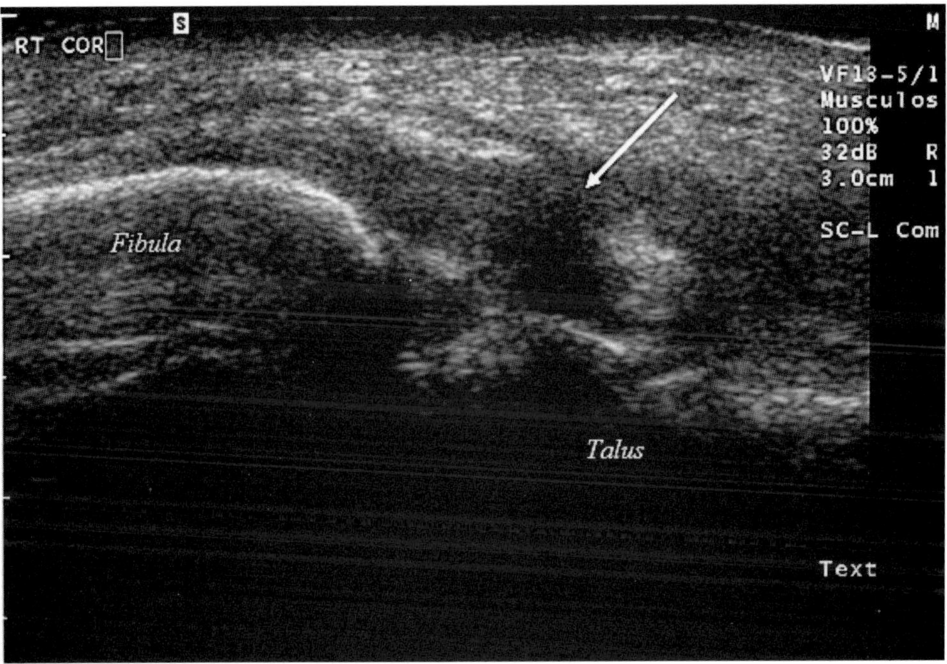

FIG. 4-30. A: Ultrasound image along the lateral aspect of the ankle demonstrates a focal tear of anterior talofibular ligament (*arrow*). Note the discontinuity of the ligament apparent as a discrete hypoechoic defect (*arrow*). **B:** Full-thickness tear (*arrow*) of the ATF in another patient.

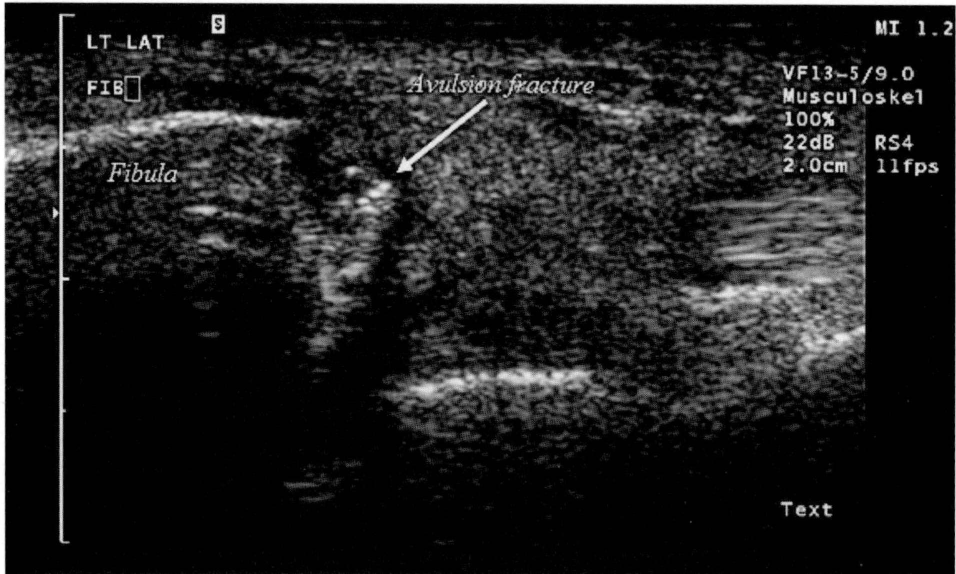

FIG. 4-31. In the setting of an inversion injury, associated avulsion fractures should be sought during real time examination. In this case, a complete tear of the ATF was demonstrated. In addition, a focal cortical avulsion of the fibula tip (*arrow*) was present.

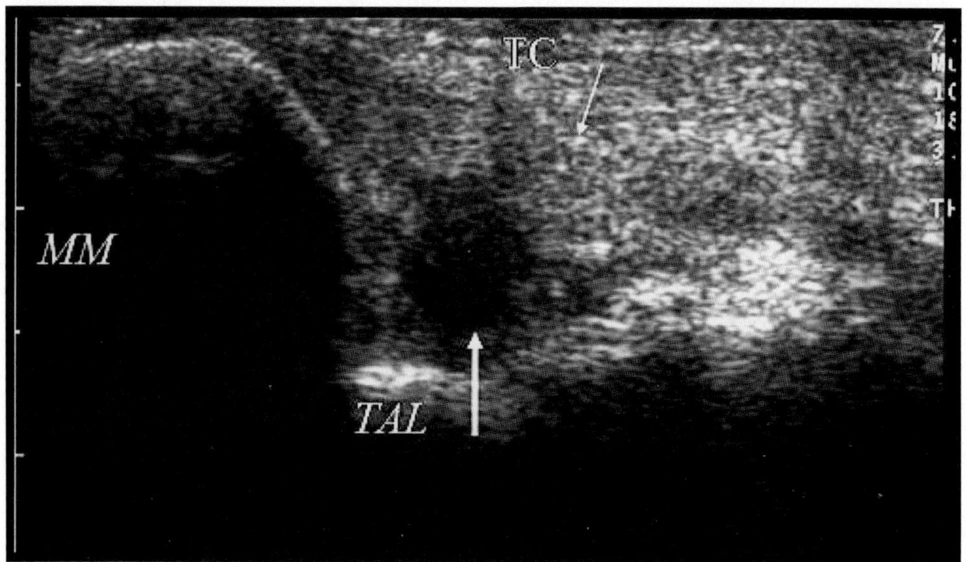

A

FIG. 4-32. A: Longitudinal image along the medial ankle demonstrates a tear of the deep fibers of the deltoid ligament (*thick white arrow*). The more superficial talocalcaneal fibers (*long white arrow*) remain in continuity. The medial malleolus (MM) and talus (TAL) are indicated.

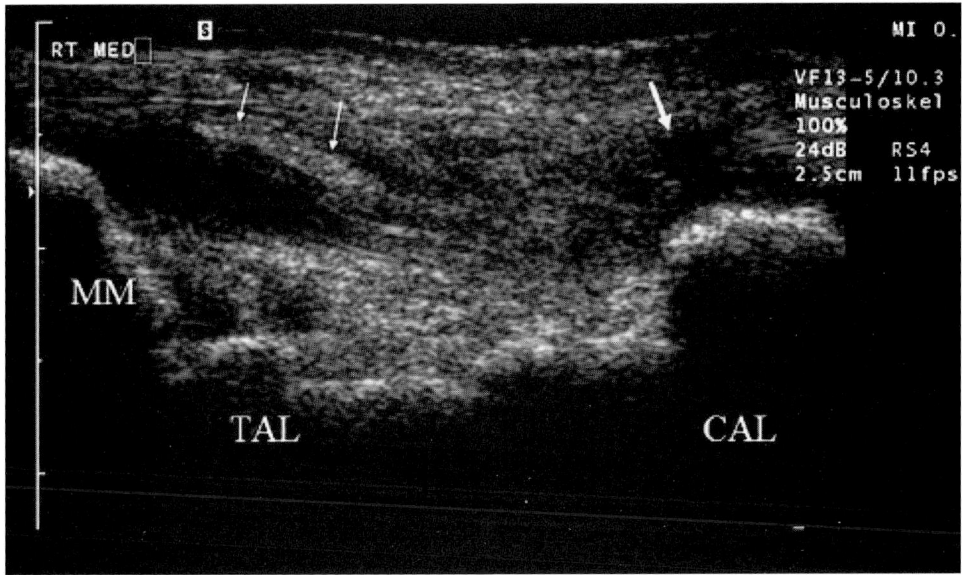

B

FIG. 4-32. B: Longitudinal image along the medial joint line demonstrates tears of the superficial (talocalcaneal) and tibionavicular fibers of the deltoid ligament (*arrows*). The medial malleolus (MM), talus (TAL), and calcaneus (CAL) are so indicated.

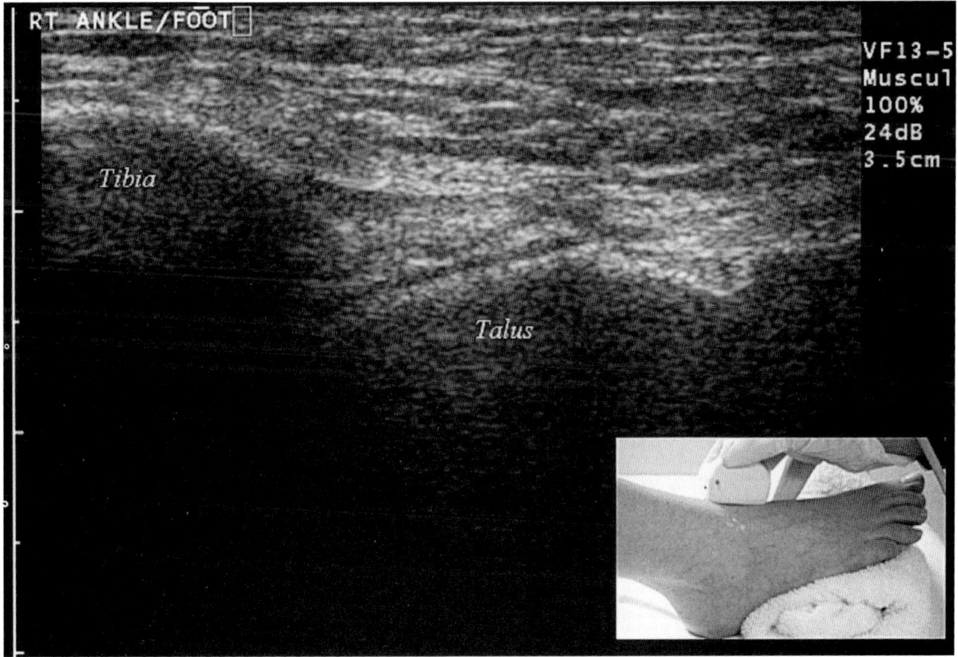

FIG. 4-33. Longitudinal ultrasound image of the tibiotalar joint. Normally, there should be little, if any, fluid in the joint. Echogenic fibroadipose tissue should fill the anterior recess, as in this case. Note the thin hypoechoic line overlying the talus. This corresponds to hyaline cartilage of the talar dome. The tibia is labeled.

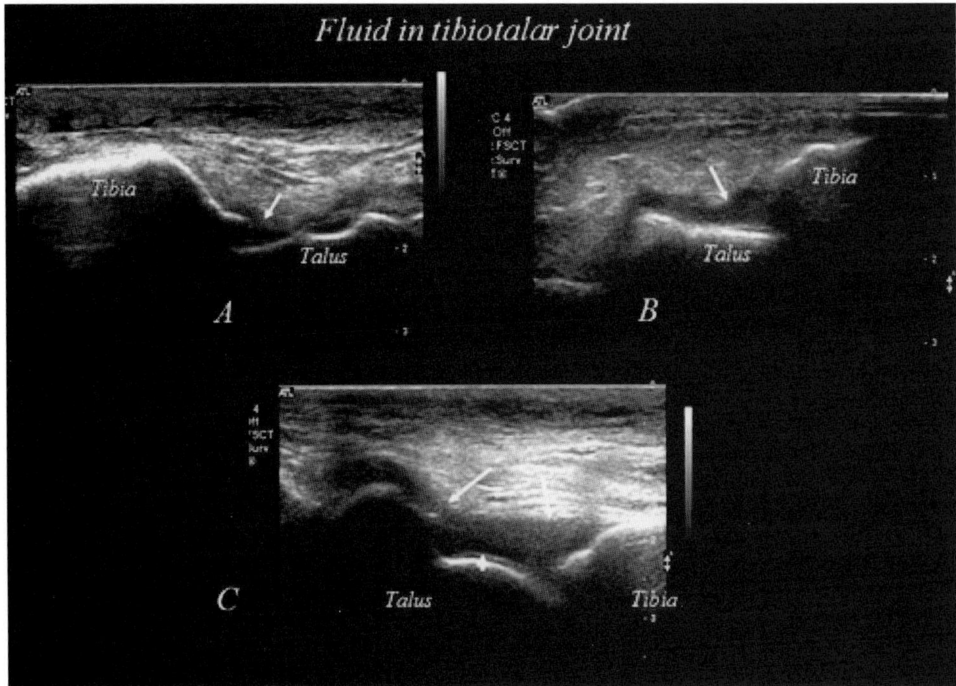

FIG. 4-34. Multiple longitudinal images of the tibiotalar joint demonstrate increasing amounts of tibiotalar joint effusion. **A:** Note a small amount of hypoechoic fluid in the tibiotalar joint (*arrow*). **B:** Coned down longitudinal image demonstrating a moderate amount of fluid in the joint space. **C:** A moderate to large amount of fluid in the joint space (*long thin white arrow*). Note the interface between the joint fluid and the articular cartilage over the talar head (*short white arrow*). Complex fluid may sometimes mimic inflammatory pannus. The ability to compress the anterior recess with the transducer favors fluid, whereas the presence of blood flow on power Doppler favors soft tissue.

REFERENCES

1. Shetty M, Fessell DP, Femino JE, et al. Sonography of ankle tendon impingement with surgical correlation. *AJR Am J Roentgenol* 2002;179:949–953.
2. Jacobson JA. Ultrasound in sports medicine. *Radiol Clin North Am* 2002;40(2):363–386.
3. Milz P, Milz S, Putz R, et al. 13 MHz high-frequency sonography of the lateral ankle joint ligaments and the tibiofibular syndesmosis in anatomic specimens. *J Ultrasound Med* 1996;15:277–284.
4. Nazarian LN, Rawoll NM, Martin CE, et al. Synovial fluid in the hindfoot and ankle: detection of amount and distribution with ultrasound. *Radiol* 1995;197:275–278.
5. Fessell DP, van Holsbeeck MT. Foot and ankle sonography. *Radiol Clin North Am* 1999;37(4):831–858.

5

Hindfoot

ACHILLES TENDON AND RETROCALCANEAL BURSA

Clinical Considerations

The Achilles tendon is susceptible to injury because of its diminished blood supply, particularly after 30 years of age, when studies have demonstrated a 30% decrease in blood supply. The "weekend warrior" is more susceptible to Achilles tendon injuries owing to improper warmup and stretching and poor overall conditioning. Overuse injuries and chronic inflammation of the Achilles tendon are also important predisposing factors to partial and complete tearing. Ultrasound imaging assists the clinician to determine the exact pathology at hand. For example, retrocalcaneal bursitis may present with symptoms similar to those of acute or chronic Achilles tendinitis. Ultrasonography demonstrates a clear and distinct difference between these entities, thus permitting the clinician to address the pathology more specifically. In addition, ultrasound examination is able to detect early changes in the Achilles tendon, allowing the clinician to prevent further progression of the tendinosis and a resulting partial or complete rupture.

Ultrasound Evaluation

Achilles tendon morphology is best visualized with a high-frequency (10 MHz or higher) linear transducer. Normally, the patient is positioned prone with the foot dorsiflexed (Fig. 5-1). Images of the Achilles tendon should be obtained in the longitudinal and transverse planes, from the muscle–tendon junction to the insertion (Fig. 5-2). Extended field of view imaging aids in obtaining a broader anatomic overview of the Achilles tendon (Fig. 5-3). The entirety of the tendon can be visualized, from the myotendinous junction to the calcaneal insertion.

The tendon normally appears echogenic and fibrillar. A thin echogenic layer of surrounding connective tissue, the paratenon, envelops the tendon. The principle of anisotropy must been taken into consideration when imaging the Achilles tendon. If the transducer is not properly aligned perpendicular to the Achilles tendon, a falsely hypoechoic image of the Achilles tendon will be obtained, mimicking tendinopathy (1).

Measurements of Achilles tendon thickness should be obtained directly in the transverse plane (2). The Achilles tendon should not be greater than 5 to 6 mm in anteroposterior dimension; thicknesses greater than this may be indicative of tendinopathy (3).

The retrocalcaneal bursa normally contains minimal, if any, fluid. In the normal state, a longitudinal image of the Achilles insertion at the calcaneus should only demonstrate a triangular focus of hyperechoic fat in the retrocalcaneal bursa (see Fig. 5-2). Distention of the bursa greater than 2 to 3 mm is considered abnormal (4) (Fig. 5-4). When inflamed, the

(Text continues on page 76)

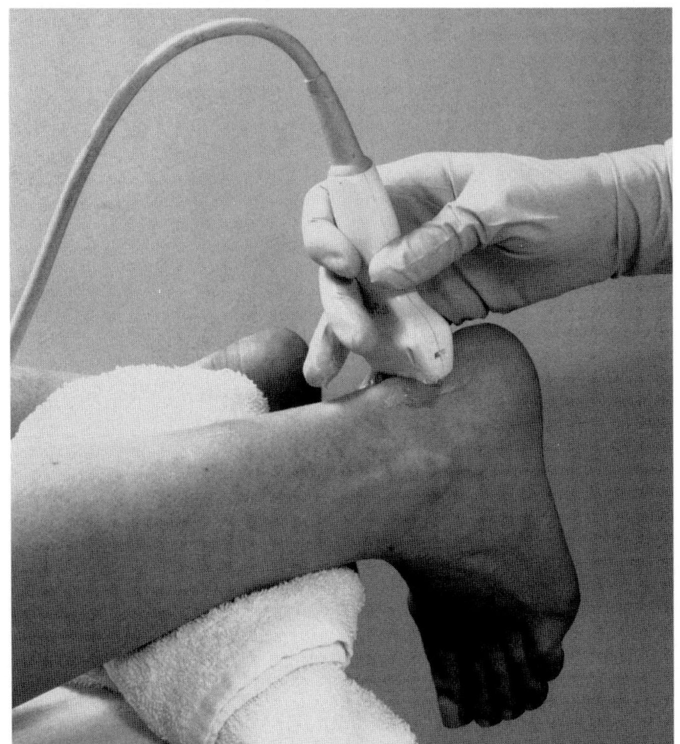

A

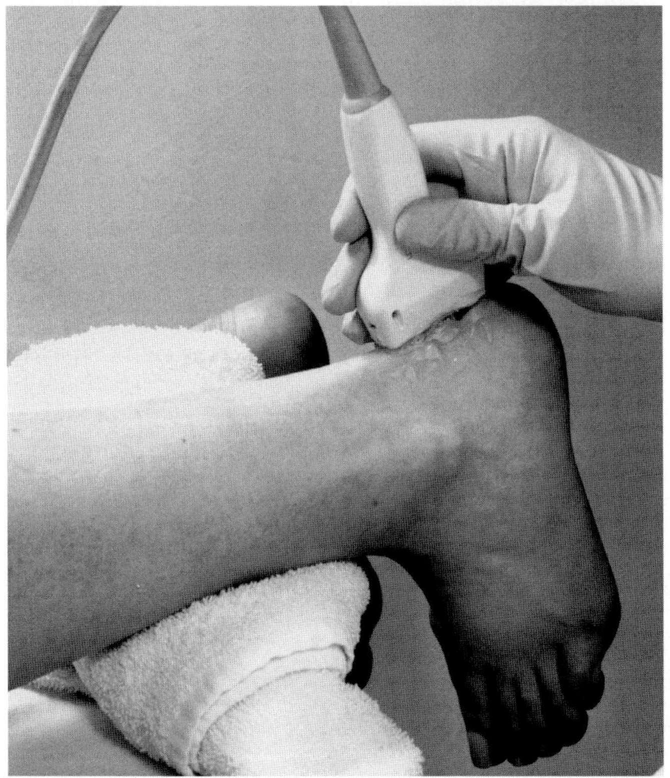

B

FIG. 5-1. A: Imaging of the Achilles tendon is performed with the patient prone and the foot dorsiflexed. This image shows proper technique for obtaining transverse images of the distal Achilles tendon. **B:** Longitudinal images of the Achilles tendon should also be obtained from the insertion, as demonstrated here, to the muscle tendon junction.

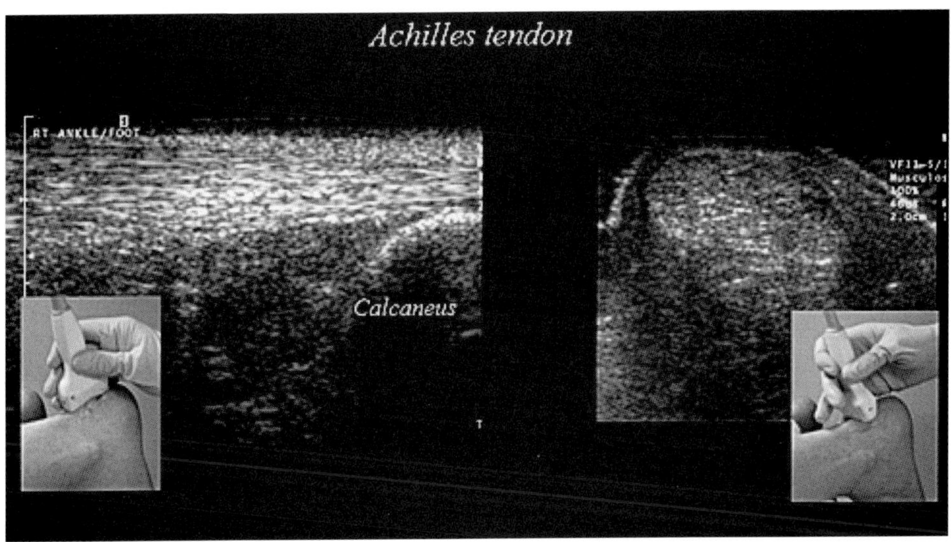

A B

FIG. 5-2. A: In long axis (**left**), the Achilles tendon is compact and fibrillar. The paratenon is closely apposed to the tendon, so that it is not readily separated from the tendon margin, as in the case of a tendon sheath. The fat deep to the tendon (Kager's fat pad) insinuates into the space between the distal tendon and calcaneus. The deep retrocalcaneal bursa is a potential space in this location. There normally should be no fluid here, although a small amount of fluid (<2 mm) should not be misinterpreted as bursitis. **B:** In short axis (**right**), the tendon appears as an echogenic ellipse, which may be difficult to separate from the adjacent fat. The tendon is best measured in this plane. The largest anteroposterior measurement should be 6 mm or less.

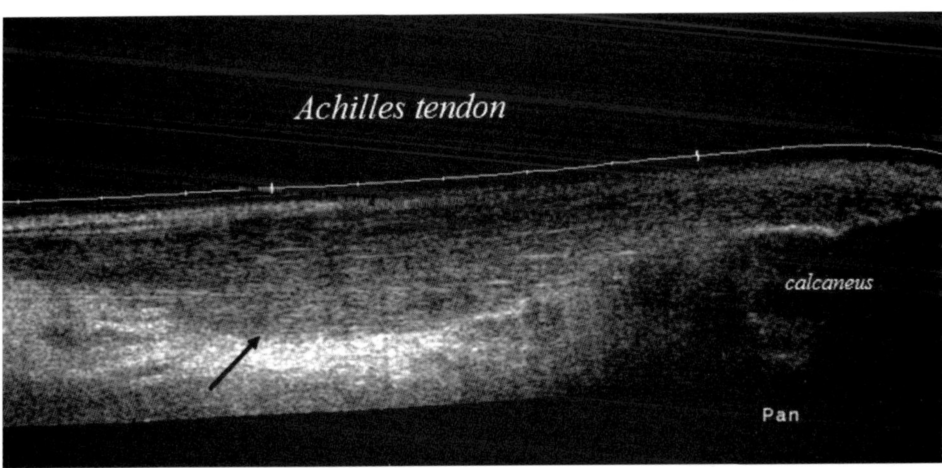

FIG. 5-3. Extended field of view imaging enables depiction of the entire length of the tendon, from the myotendinous junction to the enthesis. The full extent of tendon abnormality can be depicted in this manner. In this longitudinal extended field of view image of the Achilles tendon, there is moderate diffuse tendinosis, as demonstrated by thickening and decreased echogenicity of the Achilles tendon (*black arrow*).

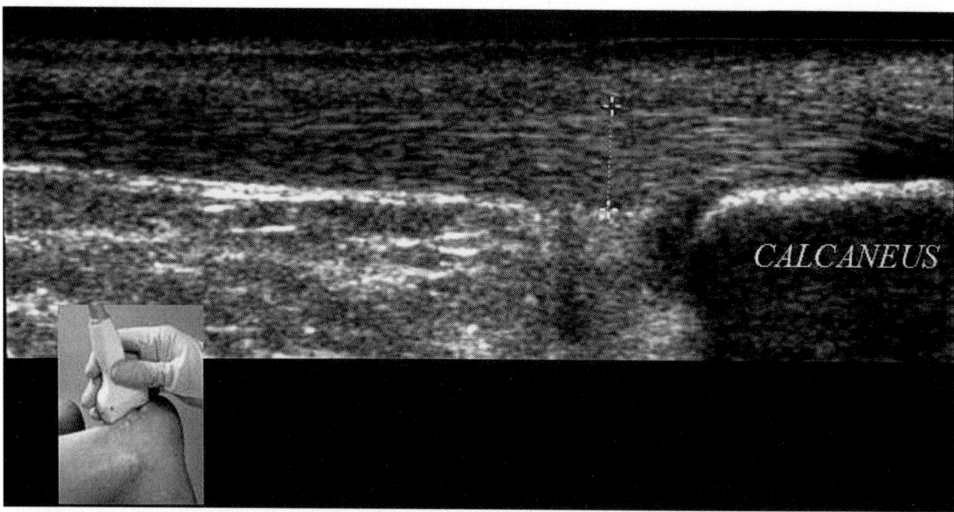

FIG. 5-4. Retrocalcaneal bursitis. Normally, no fluid or soft tissue should be seen within the deep retrocalcaneal bursa. Longitudinal image of the Achilles tendon insertion demonstrates a small amount of hypoechoic soft tissue replacing the normal fat (calcaneus labeled). The patient exhibited exquisite tenderness here and was injected under ultrasound guidance (not shown), with subsequent clinical improvement.

retrocalcaneal bursa can be distended by a moderate amount of hypoechoic fluid as well as demonstrate increased peribursal hyperemia with power Doppler (Fig. 5-5).

Tendinopathy (tendinosis, tendonitis) of the Achilles tendon is visualized as fusiform thickening of the Achilles tendon, often with decreased echogenicity (Figs. 5-3 and 5-6). Enthesopathic changes at the calcaneus can be seen during sonographic evaluation as linear or curvilinear echogenic, often shadowing, foci within the distal Achilles tendon at the enthesis (Fig. 5-7).

Tears of the Achilles tendon are demonstrated as discrete anechoic defects in the tendon, with a partial tear involving a portion of the cross-sectional diameter of the tendon and a complete tear visualized as complete tendinous discontinuity (Figs. 5-7 to 5–11). Because ultrasound is a dynamic examination, the foot can be dorsiflexed and plantar-flexed during real time evaluation, often increasing the conspicuity of a tear by visualizing widening of the tendinous gap during such provocative maneuvers (5). In the case of a proximal injury, the full gastrocnemius–soleal muscle–tendon complex should be examined in order not to miss muscle strains or discrete tears (Figs. 5-12 and 5-13). Fractures seen in association with tendon tears are not uncommon; enthesophytes may fracture, or the tendon may be weakened at the site of a dystrophic ossification (Fig. 5-9). In children, however, the growth plate is a potential weak point, and apophyseal fractures may ensue along with tendinous injury (Fig. 5-14).

Percutaneous interventions involving the retrocalcaneal bursa or Achilles paratenon can be performed using sonographic guidance (6) (Fig. 5-15). Usually, the retrocalcaneal bursa and Achilles paratenon are addressed from either a lateral or medial approach with the transducer held transversely. Once the needle tip is in the appropriate location and the steroid-

(Text continues on page 83)

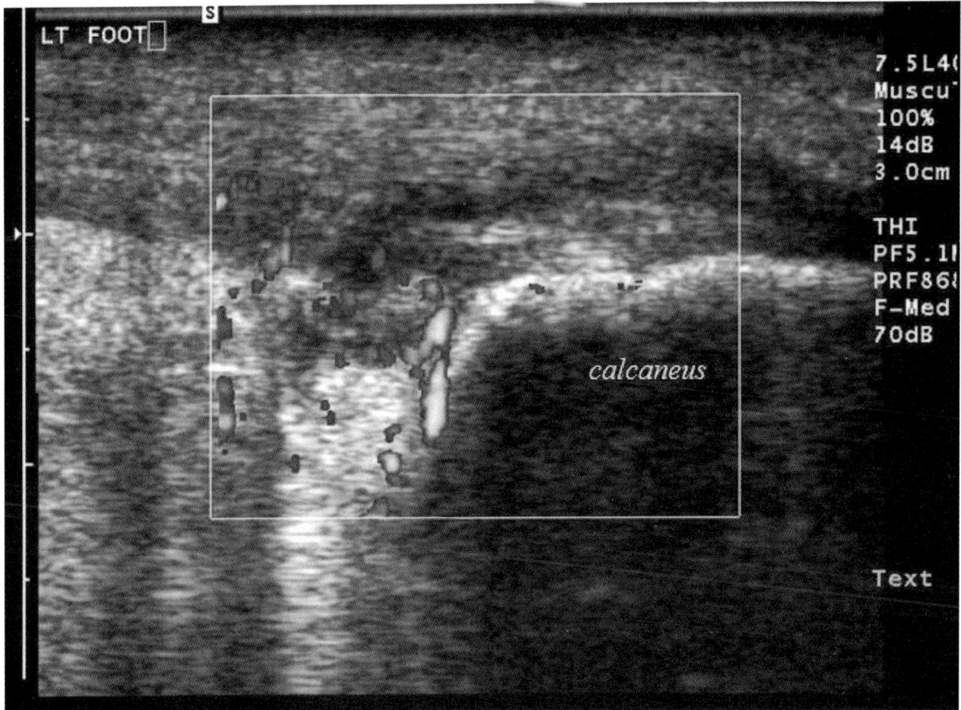

FIG. 5-5. Retrocalcaneal bursitis is often seen in association with tendon abnormalities at the enthesis. Abnormal vascularity may also be present on power Doppler imaging. In this example, marked hyperemia within the bursa extends into the deep margin of the tendon. The distal Achilles tendon is inhomogeneous with an intrasubstance split.

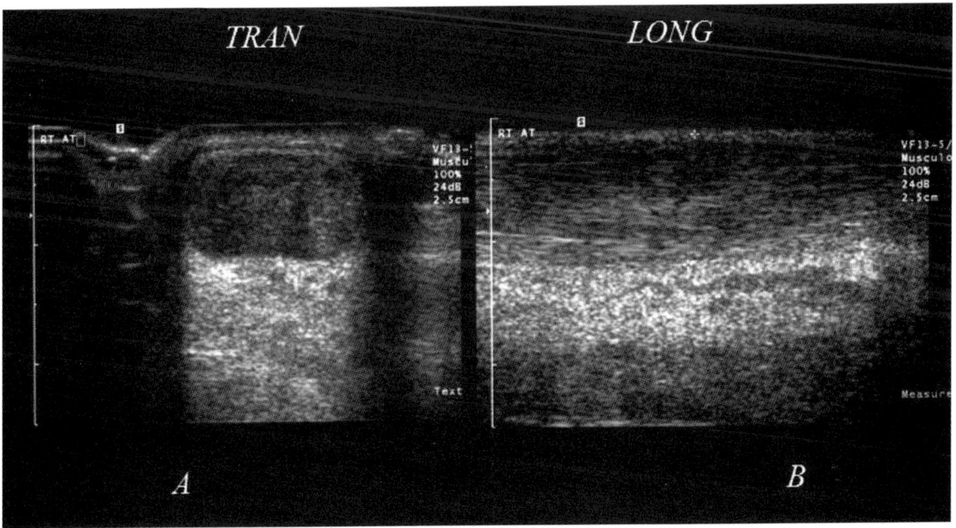

FIG. 5-6. Transverse **(A)** and longitudinal **(B)** images demonstrate Achilles tendinosis. Anteroposterior measurement of the Achilles tendon should be obtained directly from transverse images, and the Achilles tendon should measure less than 6 mm in anteroposterior dimension. In this patient with Achilles tendinosis, the transverse ultrasound image **(A)** demonstrates thickening and decreased echogenicity of the tendon. In long axis **(B)**, however, the fibrillar architecture of the tendon is still apparent.

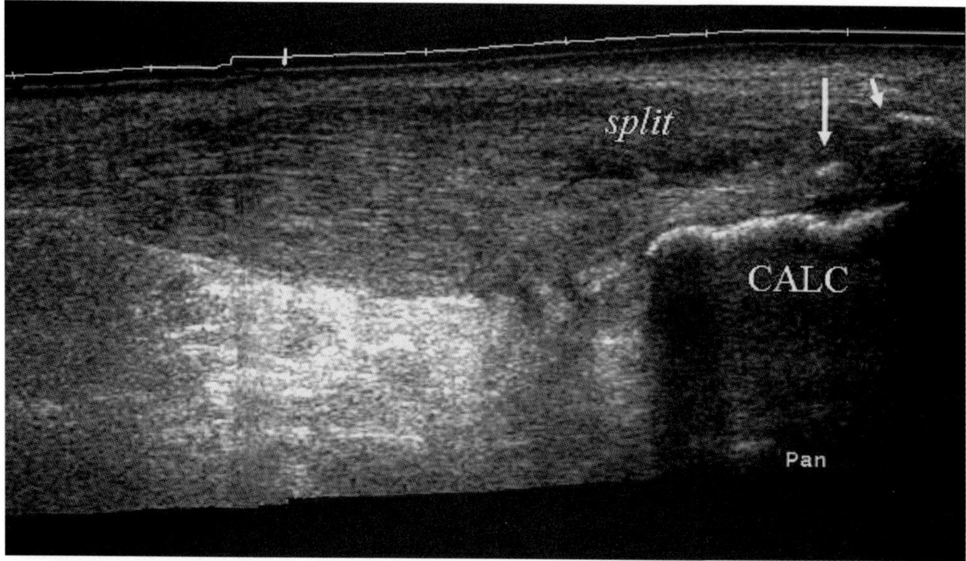

FIG. 5-7. Longitudinal extended field of view image of the Achilles tendon demonstrates diffuse tendinosis with an insertional split. Enthesopathic ossification can also be seen (*arrows*). The calcaneus (CALC) is labeled for reference.

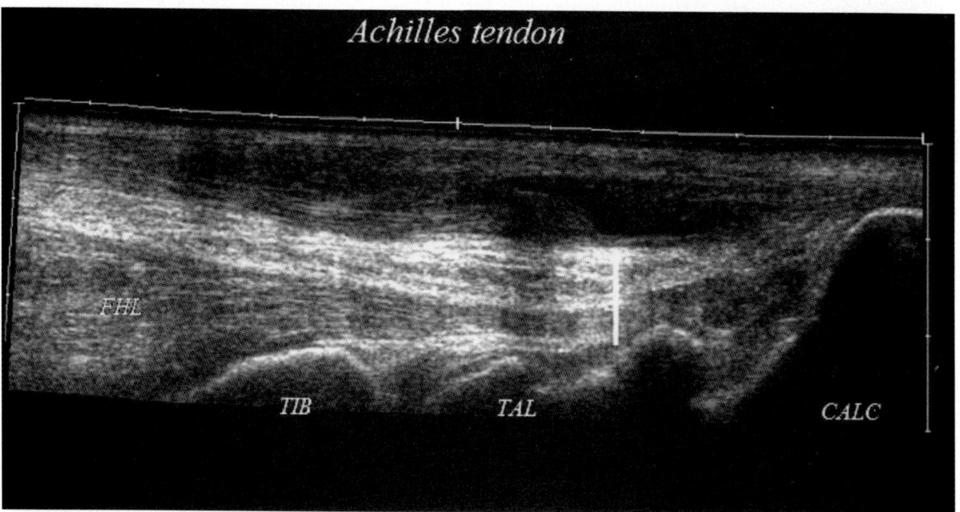

FIG. 5-8. Longitudinal extended field of view image of the Achilles tendon demonstrates advanced tendinosis with a superimposed irregular fluid-filled anechoic defect corresponding to a high-grade partial tear within the substance of tendon (*arrow*). The tibia (TIB), talus (TAL), and calcaneus (CALC) are indicated. The flexor hallucis longus muscle belly can also be identified (FHL).

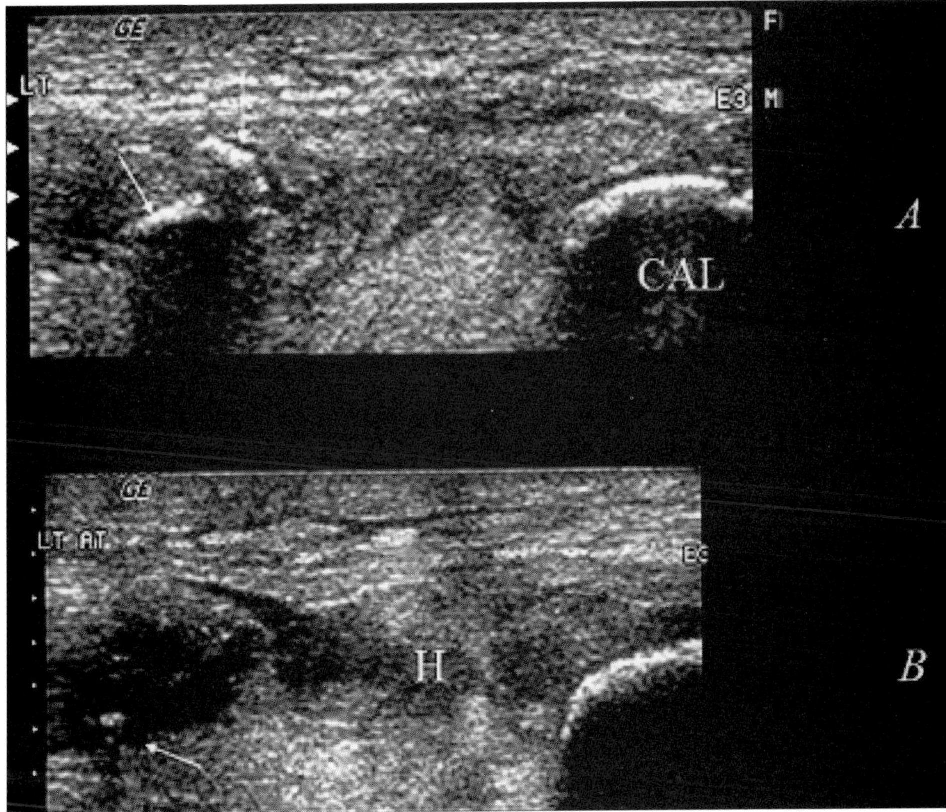

FIG. 5-9. Longitudinal images **(A, B)** demonstrate a complete tear of the Achilles tendon at the calcaneus (CAL). Small avulsion fracture fragments can be seen with the retracted tendon (*arrows*). A complex hematoma (h) replaces the tendon distally.

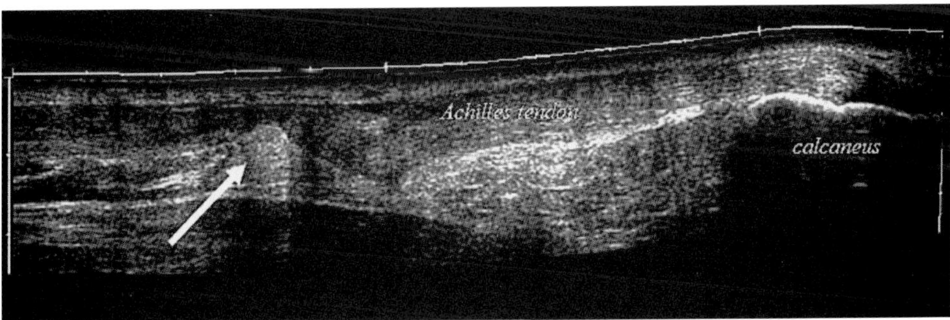

FIG. 5-10. Longitudinal extended field of view image demonstrates moderate diffuse tendinosis of the Achilles tendon with a complete muscle–tendon junction tear (*white arrow*). Note the abnormal morphology and marked attenuation of the tendon at the muscle–tendon junction. Echogenic fat herniates into the defect formed by the proximally retracted tendon.

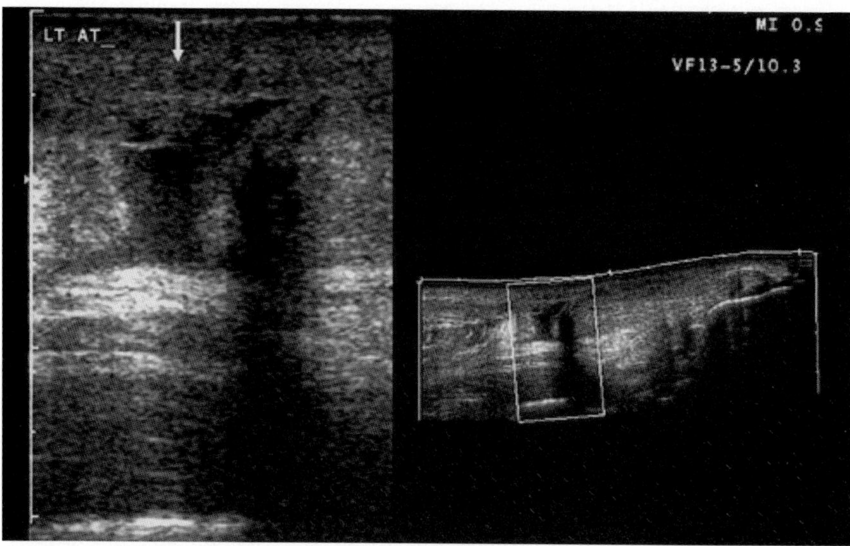

FIG. 5-11. Longitudinal extended field of view (**right**) and coned down image (**left**) of the Achilles tendon demonstrating a complete tear (*arrow*) at the myotendinous junction. A discrete hypoechoic collection is evident, resulting from the accumulation of blood in an intact paratenon. The blowup image on the left shows some intact fibers, which at surgery were shown to correspond to an intact plantaris tendon.

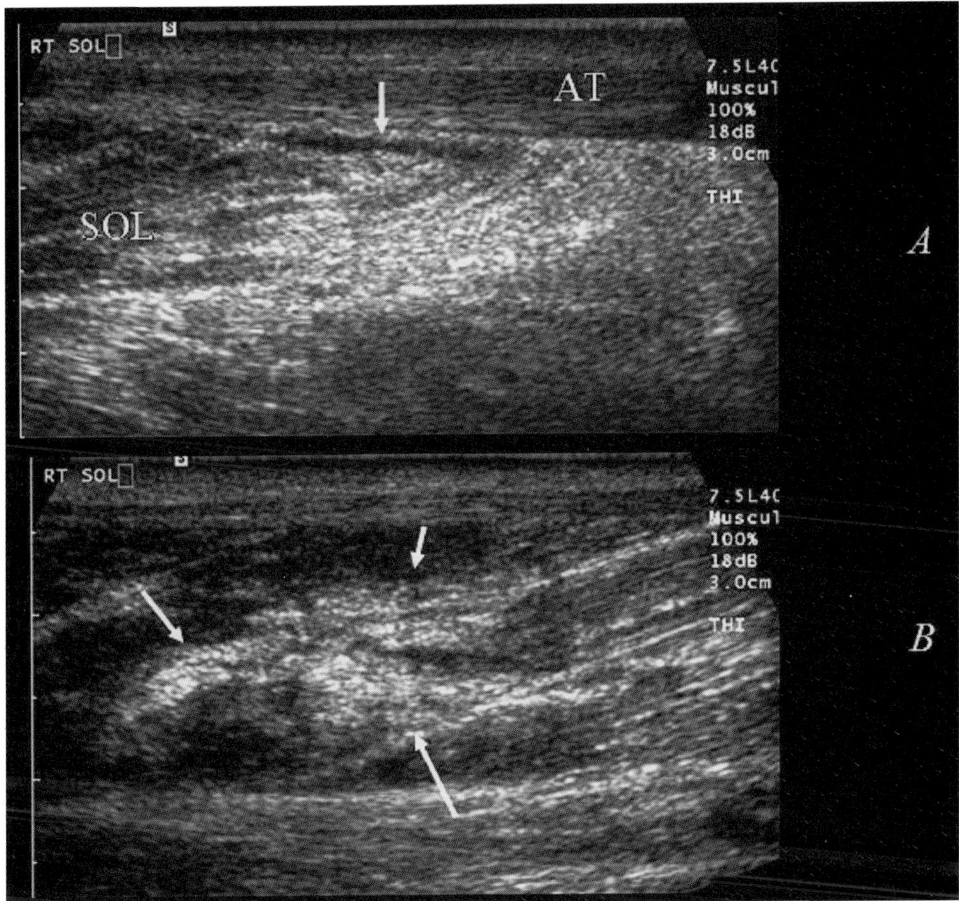

FIG. 5-12. When there is suspicion of a proximal tear, the entire muscle–tendon complex should be examined. In this case, longitudinal images of the distal soleus muscle and muscle–tendon junction demonstrate a partial muscle–tendon strain. The soleus muscle (sol) and Achilles tendon (AT) are indicated. A small amount of fluid can be seen (**A**, *arrow*) as well as hyperechoic regional intramuscular edema (**B**, *arrow*). No tear could be demonstrated in the Achilles tendon.

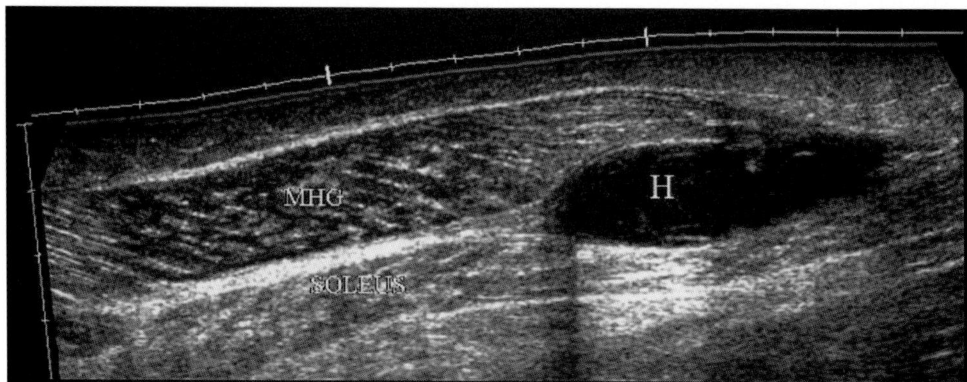

FIG. 5-13. Longitudinal extended field of view image demonstrating a large hematoma (H) at the myofascial attachment of the medial head of the gastrocnemius (MHG) and soleus muscles (also called *tennis leg*). The hematoma was aspirated under ultrasound guidance (not shown).

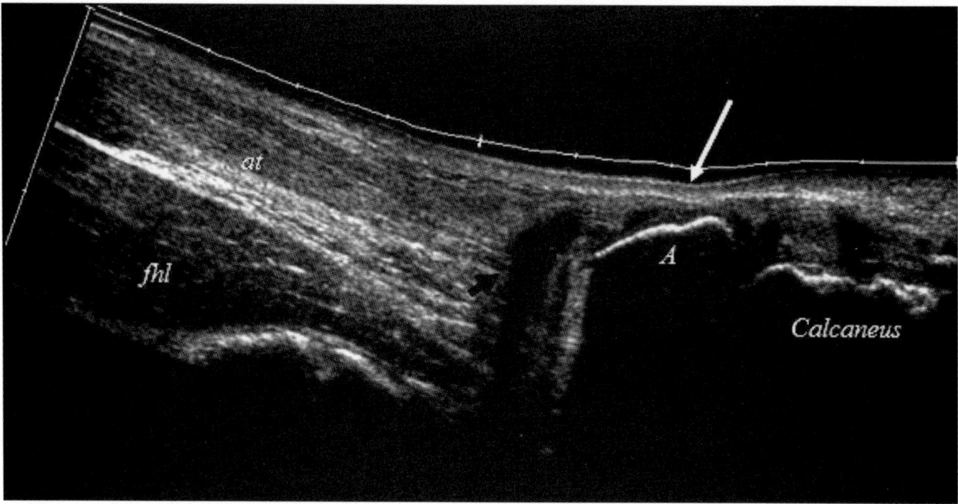

FIG. 5-14. Longitudinal extended field of view image in an adolescent with ankle pain and swelling following a "hard landing" during gymnastics. There is a moderately displaced fracture of the calcaneal apophysis (**A**, *arrow*). Moreover, a tear at the Achilles tendon (AT) insertion can be seen (*short black arrow*) and distal to the apophyseal fragment. The flexor hallucis long (fhl) and calcaneus are labeled for reference.

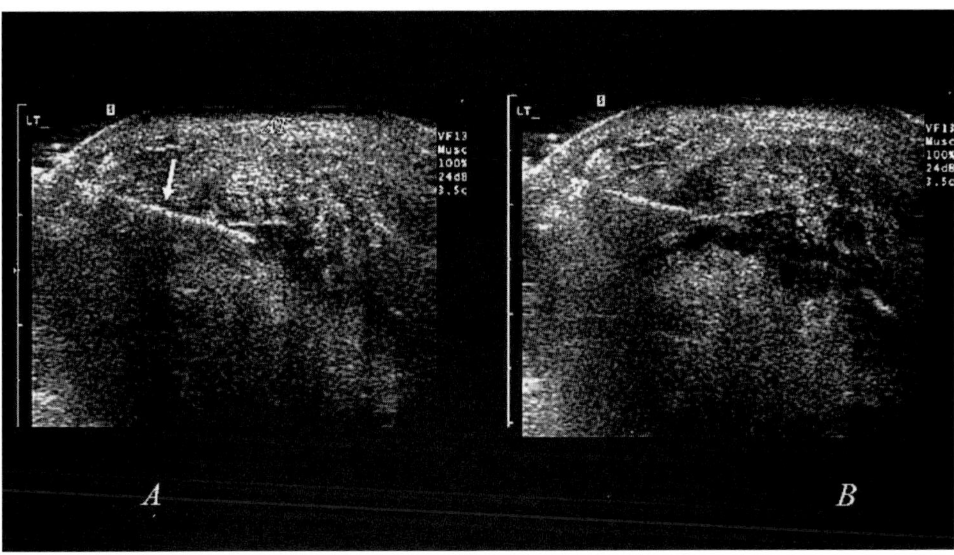

FIG. 5-15. Typically, the retrocalcaneal bursa and Achilles paratenon are injected from a short axis approach. The needle tip enters the skin either from a medial or lateral approach, as demonstrated here. In this case **(A)**, a 25-gauge needle (*arrow*) is placed into the deep retrocalcaneal bursa. During real time observation, the bursa is distended **(B)** with a steroid-anesthetic mixture. Ultrasound enables one to monitor needle position and distribution of the therapeutic mixture.

anesthetic mixture is instilled, one can turn the transducer 90 degrees to visualize the bursa distend with fluid or visualize fluid tracking along the Achilles paratenon.

Infiltrative abnormalities of the Achilles tendon are uncommon, although certain abnormalities have a predilection for extensor surfaces, such as gout (Figs. 5-16 and 5–17; see also Chapter 2) or tendon xanthomas. Tophaceous deposition is typically echogenic and may be difficult to separate from adjacent fibrofatty connective tissue. The presence of hyperemia may be of value in demonstrating the secondary inflammatory reaction produced as a result.

PLANTAR FASCIA

Clinical Considerations

Ultrasound is invaluable in assessing the extent of damage to the plantar fascia. Patients are often diagnosed clinically with heel spur syndrome and plantar fasciitis. Ultrasound often demonstrates the presence of a tear in the fascia that will change the treatment options to be more aggressive in nature. Ultrasound evaluation is very useful in identifying calcaneal fat pad injuries, which are often misdiagnosed as plantar fasciitis. We believe that a patient presenting with heel pain should have a baseline ultrasound examination in addition to radiographs. The results of both examinations should be integrated and used to design and select treatment options.

All too often, a patient is treated for plantar fasciitis that does not respond to any of the recommended and available treatment options. In many of these cases, the patient was treated for a condition that was not present. A plantar fibroma is often clinically confused with plantar fasciitis and therefore not treated adequately. Ultrasound distinguishes between the two conditions and further assists the clinician to select the appropriate treatment.

(Text continues on page 86)

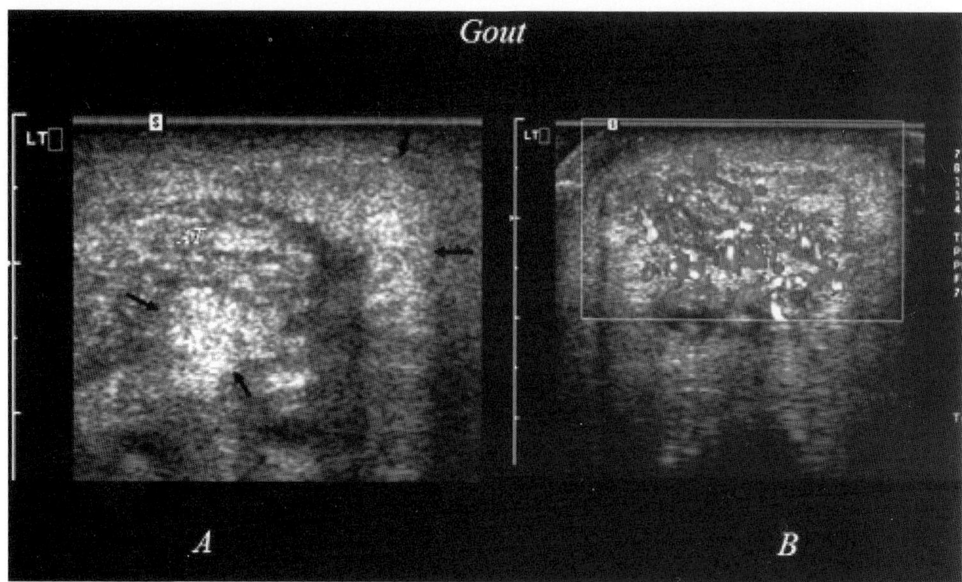

FIG. 5-16. Power Doppler imaging provides a useful clinical adjunct in evaluation of inflammatory arthropathies. **A:** Gray scale transverse image of the Achilles tendon (**left,** AT) demonstrates small, nodular echogenic foci about the tendon (*black arrows*). **B:** Application of power Doppler demonstrates marked regional hyperemia consistent with inflammation. The small echogenic foci are tophaceous deposits in this patient with gout.

C

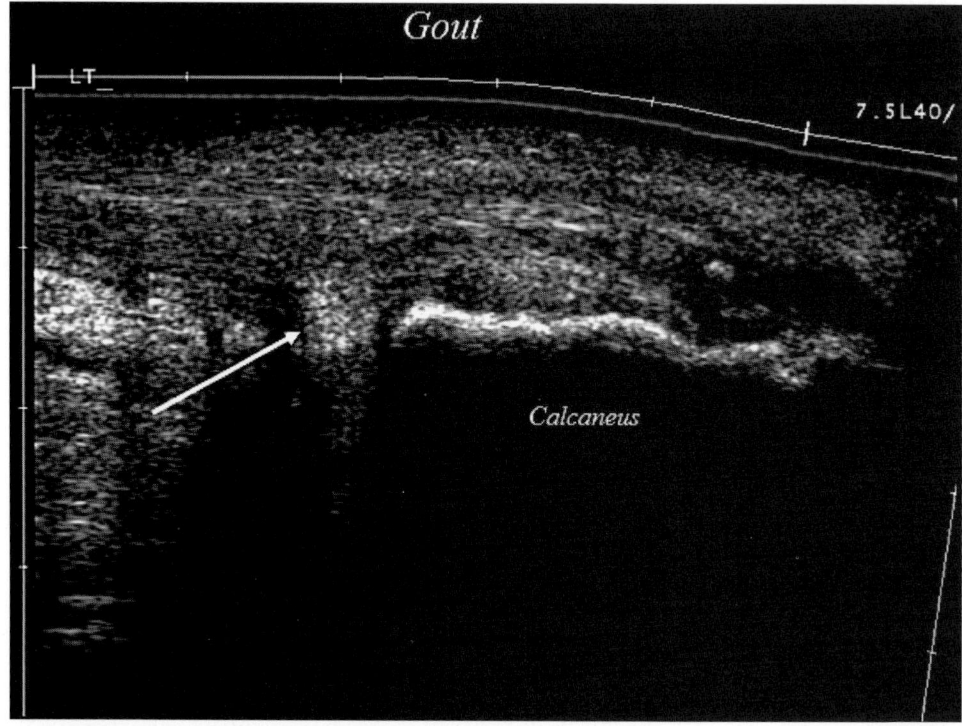

C: Longitudinal extended field of view image in the same patient demonstrating an echogenic tophus (*arrow*) in the retrocalcaneal bursal region. Enthesopathic tendinosis is present at the calcaneus.

A

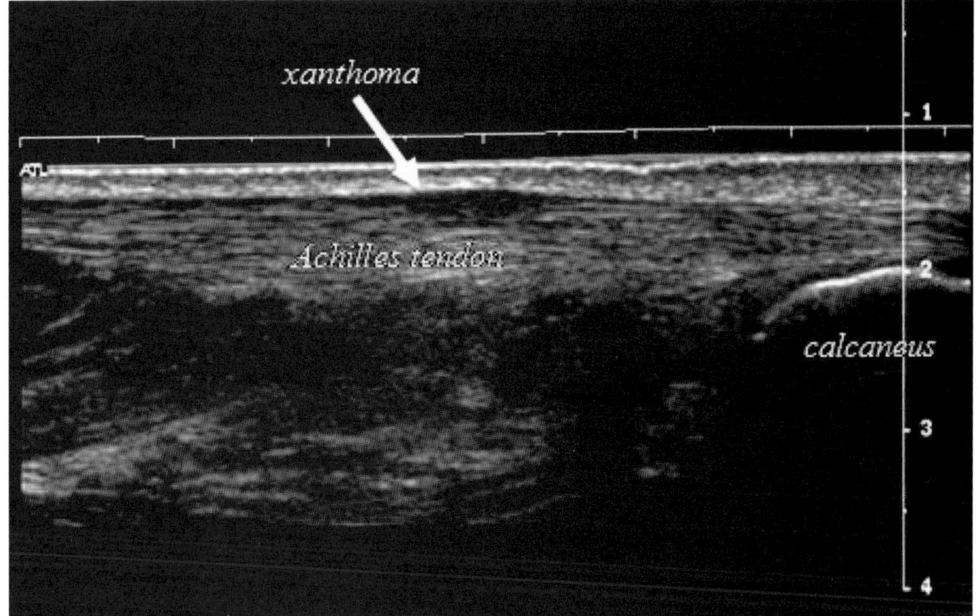

B

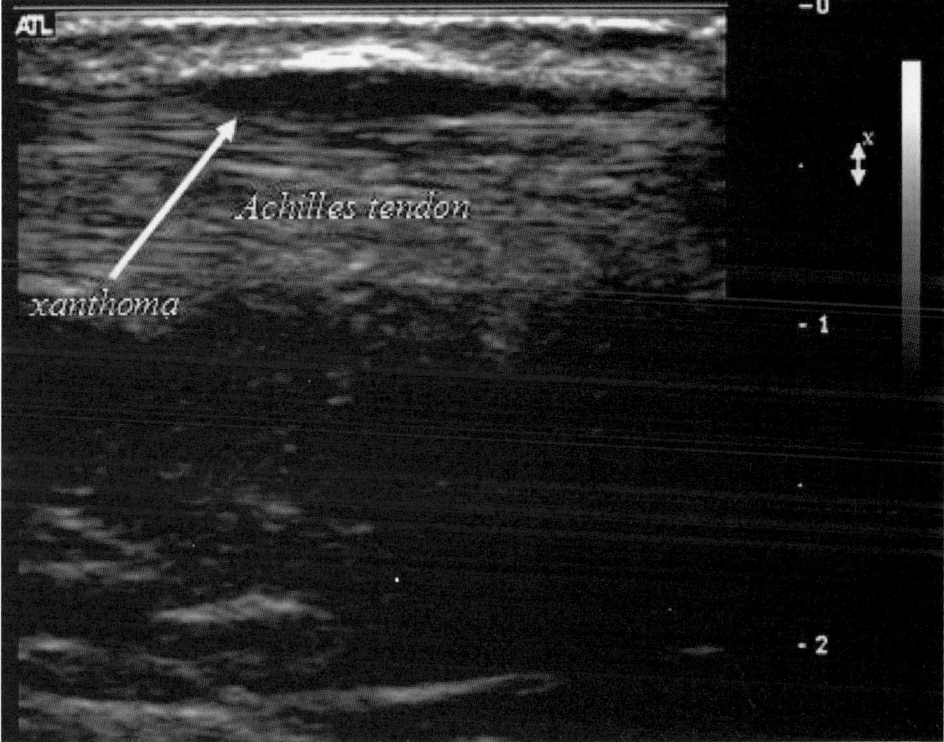

FIG. 5-17. Ultrasound has been shown to be a sensitive technique to detect tendon xanthomas. In patients with the heterozygous form of familial hypercholesterolemia, Achilles xanthomas are an important diagnostic feature of the disease. **A:** This longitudinal extended field of view image of the distal Achilles tendon demonstrates a hypoechoic nodule within the superficial margin of the tendon. The patient had a history of hypercholesterolemia, with a parent and sibling having died from coronary artery disease. **B:** The xanthoma is better depicted in this small field of view gray scale image. Typically, these are hypoechoic and oriented along the long axis of the tendon. With advanced disease, the xanthomas may become confluent and difficult to differentiate from tendinosis.

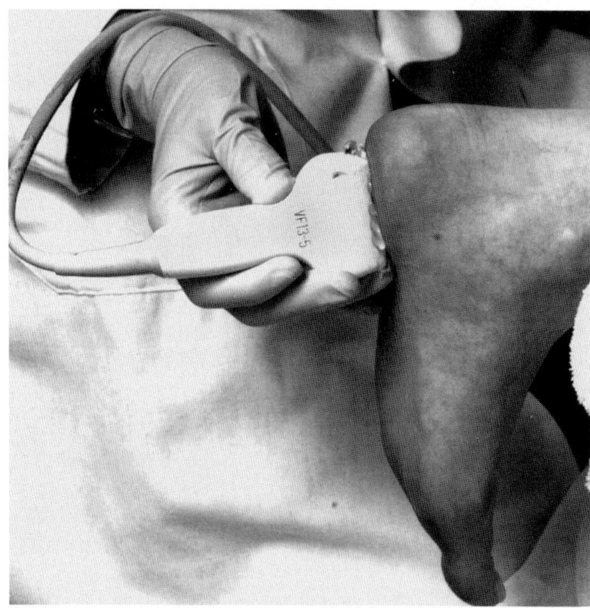

FIG. 5-18. The plantar fascia is typically imaged with the patient prone and the foot dorsiflexed. The plantar fascia should be evaluated at the calcaneal origin, where most pathology occurs.

Ultrasound Evaluation

The plantar fascia is best visualized with a medium-frequency (7.5 MHz) linear probe. The patient is placed prone with the foot dorsiflexed (Fig. 5-18). The plantar fascia should be imaged from the calcaneus to the mid-forefoot, especially the medial fibers. Normally, the plantar fascia is seen as a thin hyperechoic band of tissue, measuring no more than 4 mm (Fig. 5-19).

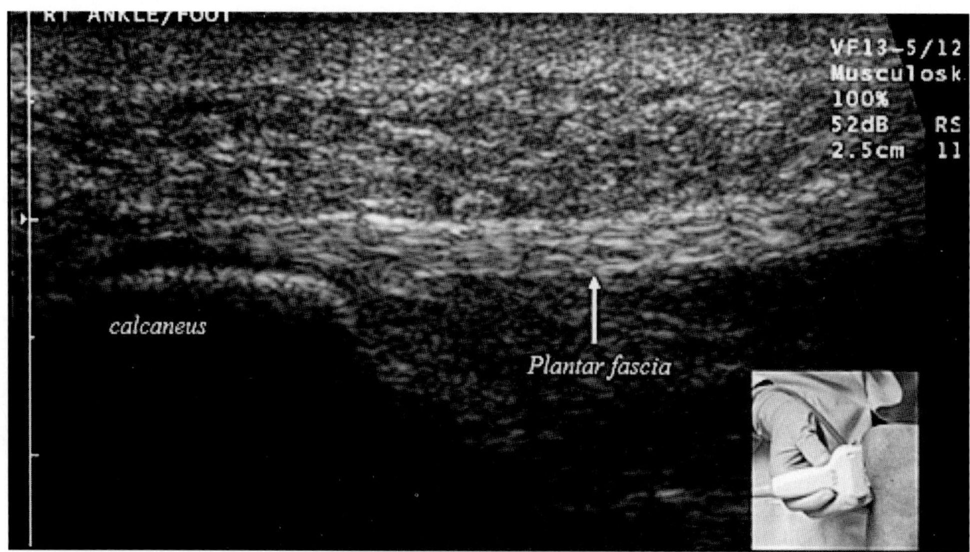

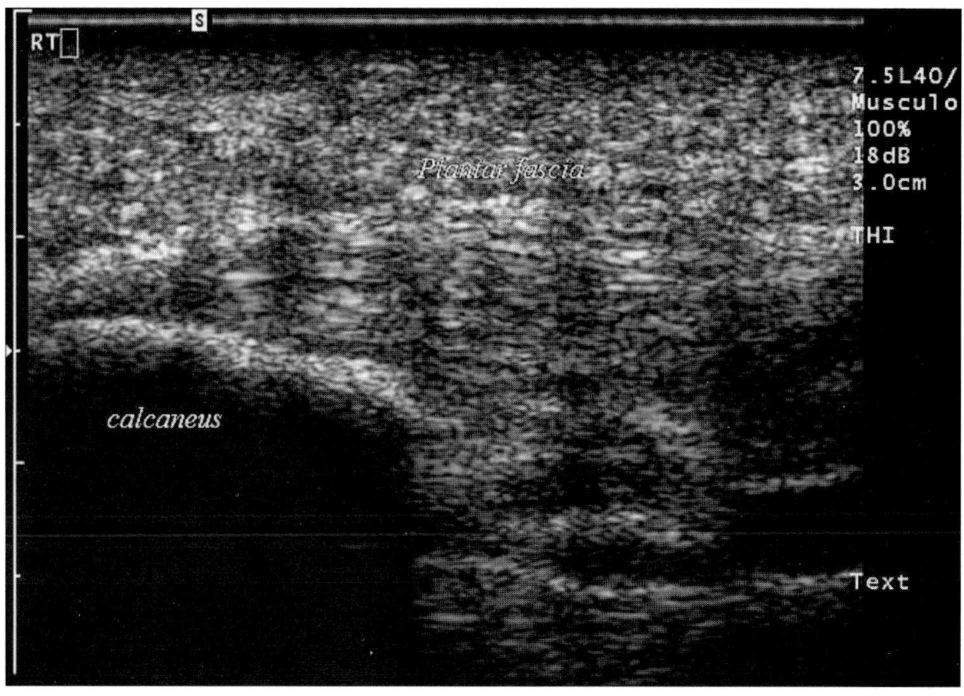

A

FIG. 5-20. Varying presentations of plantar fasciitis. **A:** Longitudinal image of the plantar fascia demonstrates mild plantar fasciitis. There is thickening and decreased echogenicity of the plantar fascia at calcaneus. Normally, the plantar fascia should measure less than 4 mm at the calcaneal orgin. Note the presence of a small spur along the base of the calcaneus.

FIG. 5-20. *(Continued on next page)*

Plantar fasciitis can be diagnosed by thickening (>4 mm) and decreased echogenicity of the plantar fascia, often with areas of more focal decreased echogenicity representing areas of cystic degeneration (7) (Fig. 5-20). Newer ultrasound technologies such as tissue harmonic imaging can aid in increasing the conspicuity of small areas of cystic degeneration. Thickening and edema of the superficial (plantar) heel fat pad can also be seen (Fig. 5-21). Tears of the plantar fascia are seen as focal fluid-filled defects in the plantar fascia with interruption in the normal fibrillar architecture. As with tendon tears, tears of the plantar fascia may be entirely intrasubstance and of partial thickness, arising from the deep or superficial margin, or they may achieve full thickness (Fig. 5-22).

Plantar fibromas are not an uncommon cause of plantar foot pain. These can be seen with sonography as either well-defined or sometimes moderately infiltrative heteroge-

(Text continues on page 92)

FIG. 5-19. Normal sonographic appearance of the plantar fascia. The plantar fascia is seen as a hyperechoic band of tissue containing fine internal fibrillar architecture, originating from the medial tubercle of the calcaneus. Normally, the plantar fascia is of uniform thickness, typically measuring about 4 mm in thickness. The plantar aspect of the calcaneus is normally smooth with a rounded margin.

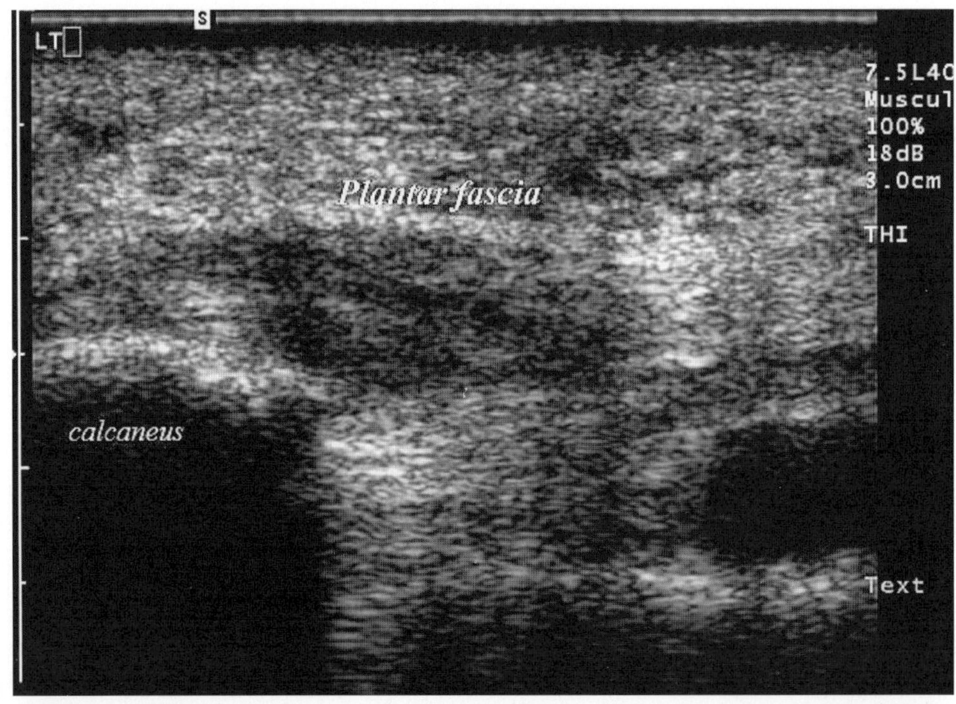

B

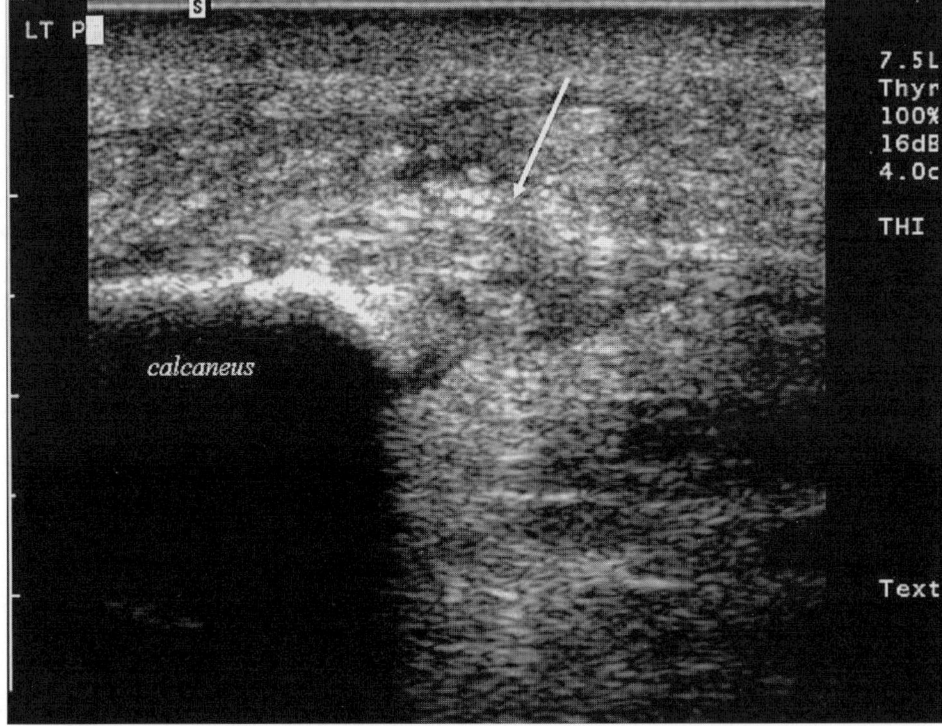

C

FIG. 5-20. B: Longitudinal ultrasound image demonstrates thickening and decreased echogenicity of the proximal plantar fascia. **C:** Longitudinal ultrasound image demonstrates thickening and deep surface fissures. Note the presence of mild reactive edema in the overlying fat pad.

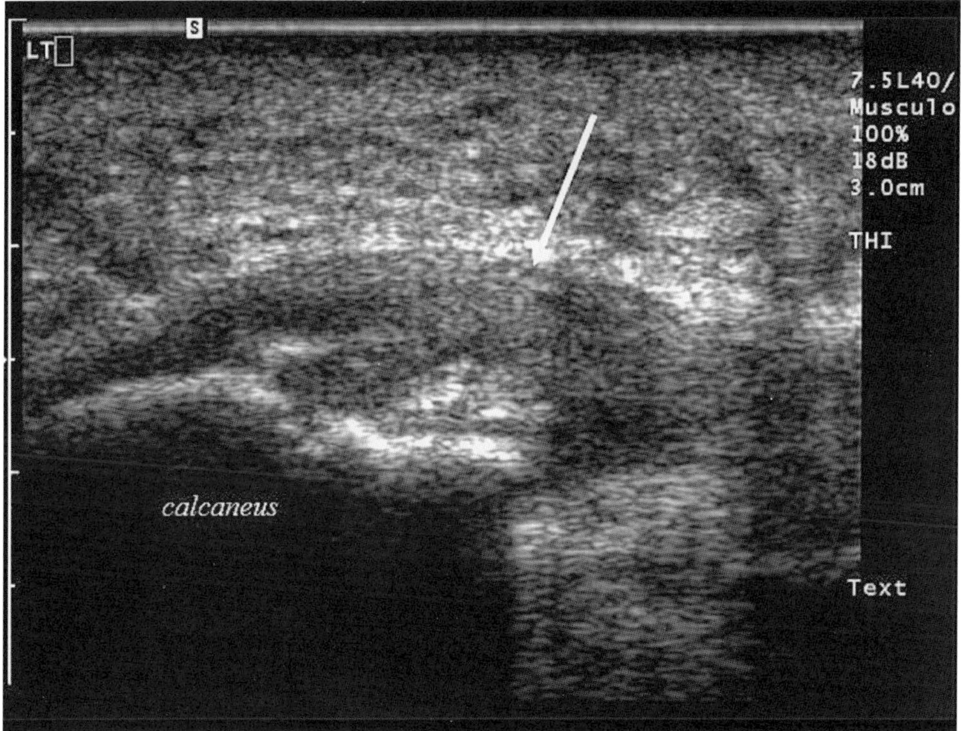

D

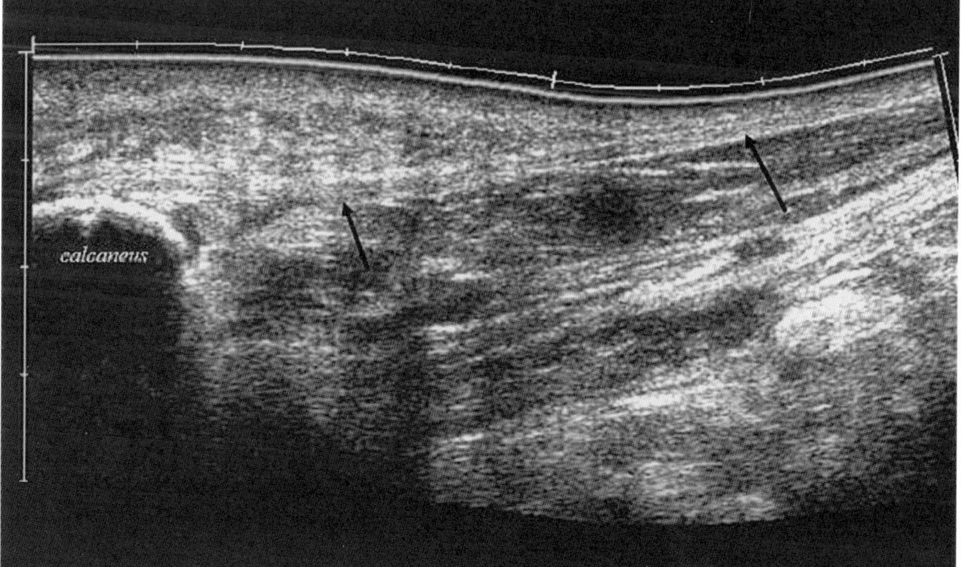

E

FIG. 5-20. D: In this case, the plantar fascia is markedly enlarged and diffusely hypoechoic with remodeling of the calcaneus. **E:** Longitudinal extended field of view image of the plantar fascia demonstrates moderate plantar fasciitis, with diffused thickening and decreased echogenicity of the proximal plantar fascia. These cases illustrate that most cases of isolated plantar fasciitis are confined to the proximal 2 to 3 cm of the plantar fascia. The distal plantar fascia (*arrows*) retains normal thickness and morphology.

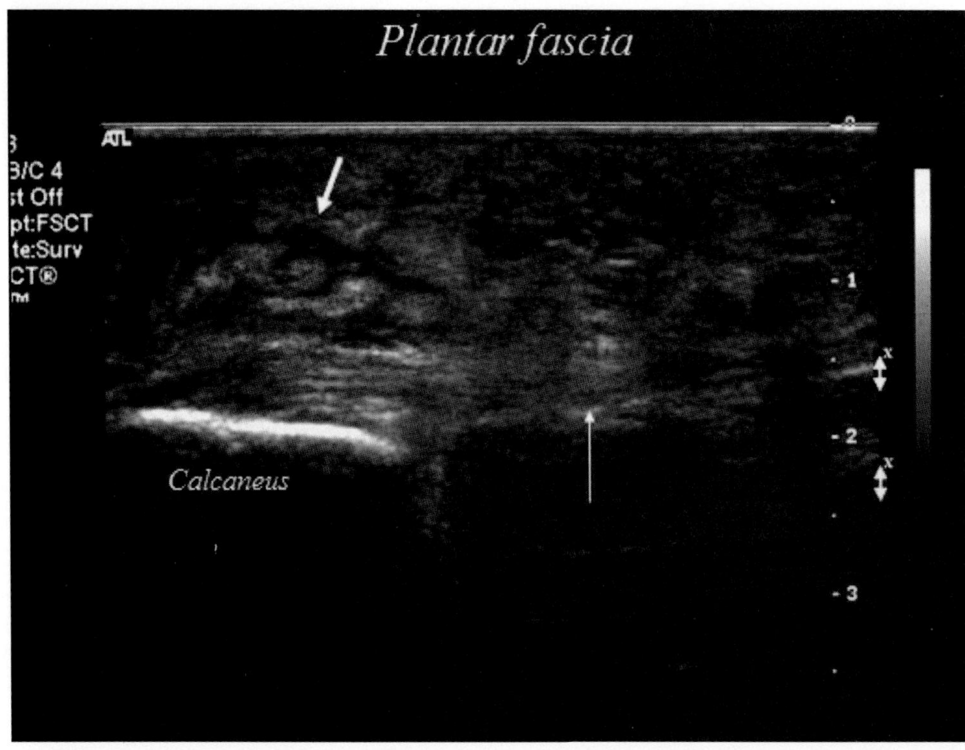

FIG. 5-21. Edema in the fat pad overlying the plantar fascia often presents as a concomitant finding seen in association with plantar fasciitis. In this case, there is striking edema (*thick arrow*) in the fat pad overlying the abnormal plantar fascia (*thin arrow*).

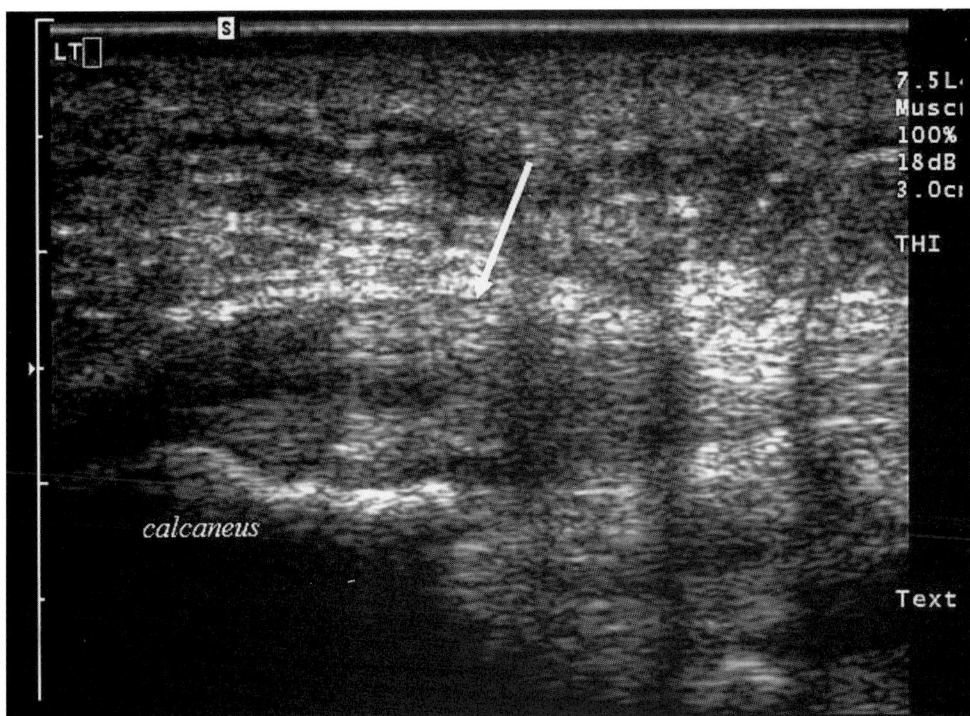

A

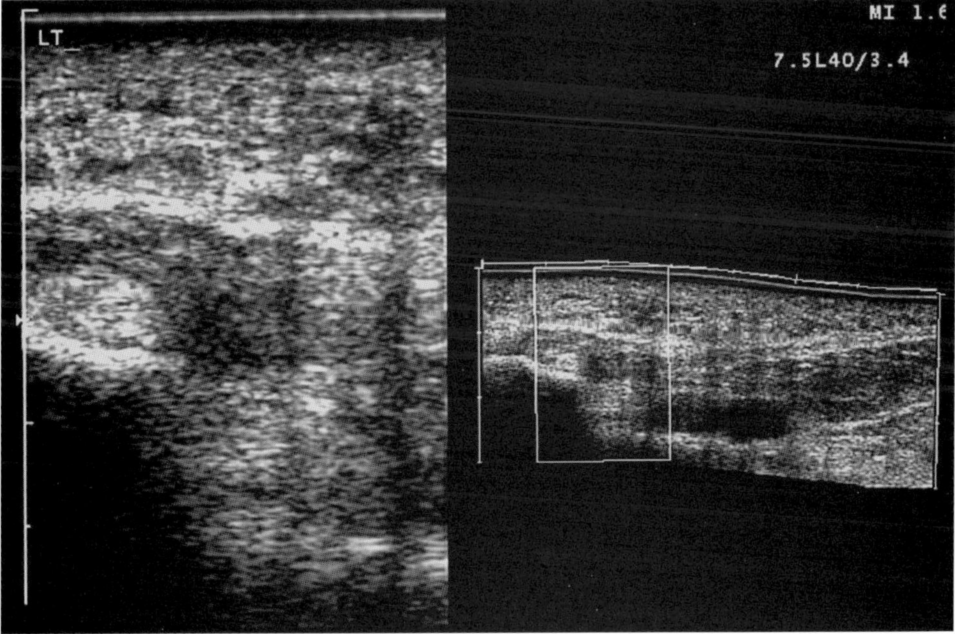

B

FIG. 5-22. Tears of the plantar fascia. These may occur in association with plantar fasciitis, as a result of trauma or iatrogenically, through a misplaced cortisone injection. **A:** In this patient with plantar fasciitis, a well-marginated hypoechoic split is seen within the fascia, representing an intrasubstance tear. **B:** More commonly, tears appear as discretely marginated defects along the deep surface of the plantar fascia, near the calcaneal margin.

FIG. 5-22. *(Continued on next page)*

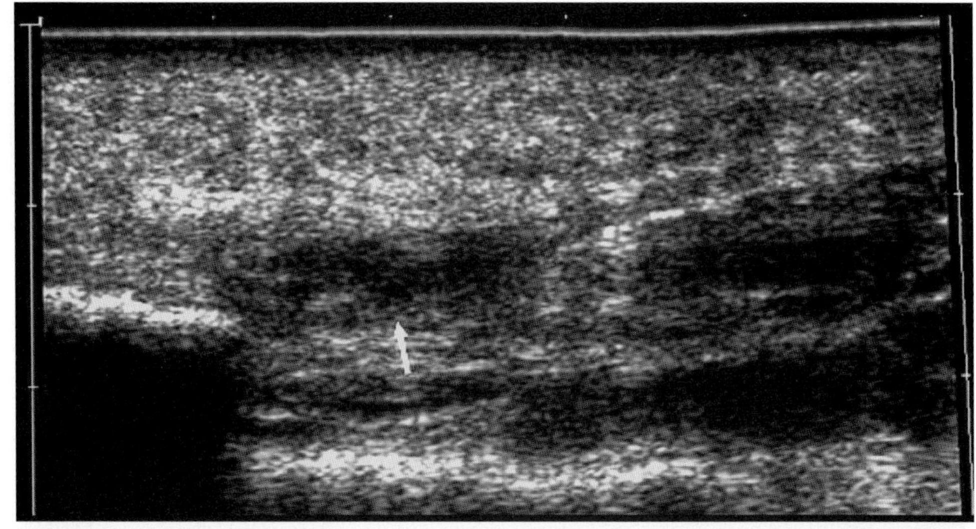

C

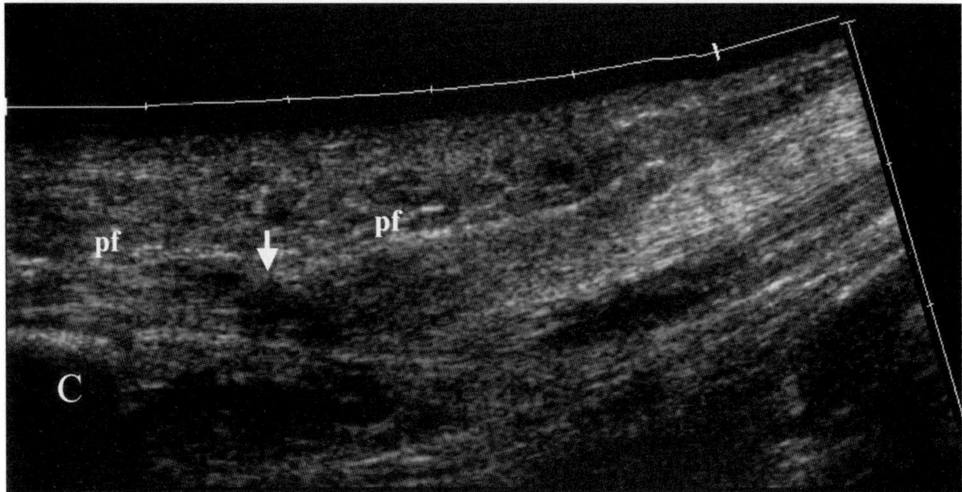

D

FIG. 5-22. C: This patient is a professional dancer who experienced sudden onset of plantar pain during rehearsal. A partial-thickness deep surface tear is present (*arrow*). **D:** Longitudinal extended field of view image in a patient with heel pain and difficulty walking following a blind cortisone injection. There is complete rupture of the plantar fascia (*arrow*). Blind cortisone injections can result in intrafascial deposition and have been associated with plantar fascia rupture.

neously hypoechoic masses along the plantar margin of the foot (Fig. 5-23). In our experience, most are found within 2 to 3 cm of the plantar fascia orgin. These are usually single lesions, but on occasion, they may be quite extensive and multiple (8,9) (Fig. 5-24).

Steroid injections directly into the plantar fascia can be associated with degeneration and ultimate rupture of the plantar fascia (10). With ultrasound, one can guide a needle in a perifascial location, infiltrating steroid and anesthetic into the heel fat pad, as opposed to directly into the plantar fascia, thus affording symptomatic relief without the theoretic risk for plantar fascia rupture.

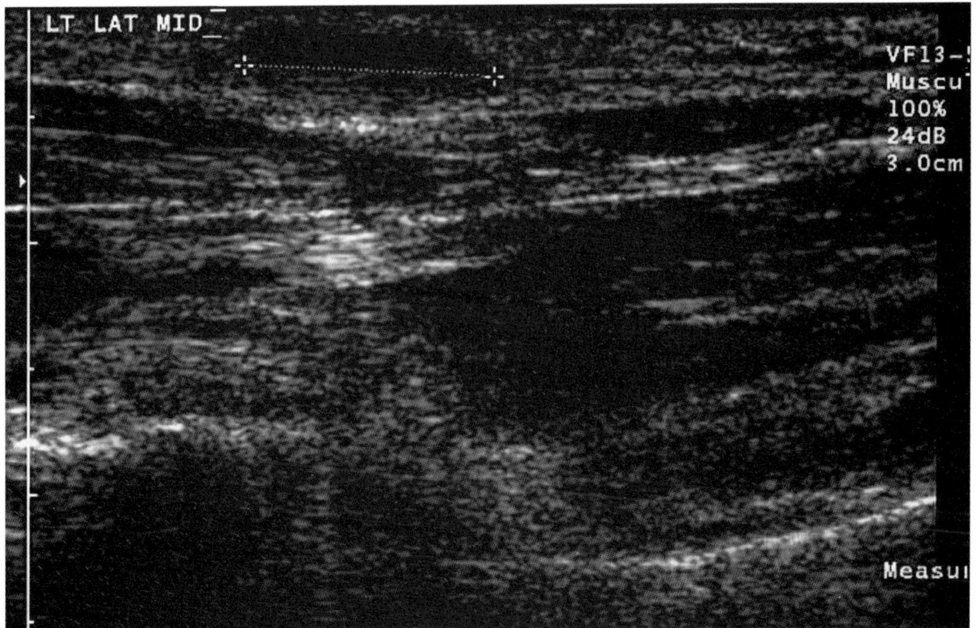

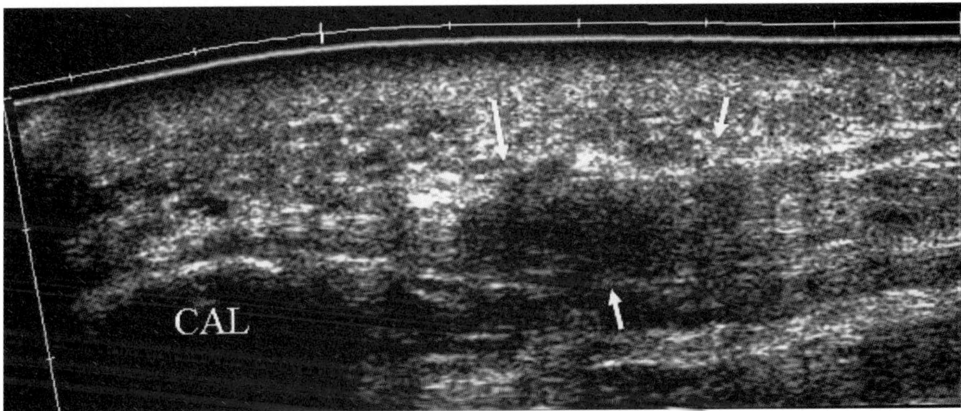

FIG. 5-23. A: Plantar fibromas present as hard palpable nodules along the plantar aspect of the foot and distal to the orgin of the plantar fascia (usually >2–3 cm). Sonographically, these appear as hypoechoic nodules oriented along the fascial axis and often arising from the superficial margin. **B:** This longitudinal extended field of view image at the level of the midfoot demonstrates fusiform dilatation of the plantar fascia, with replacement of the normally thin hyperechoic plantar fascia fibers with a hypoechoic heterogeneous mass, consistent with a plantar fibroma. Note that the origin of the plantar fascia is normal.

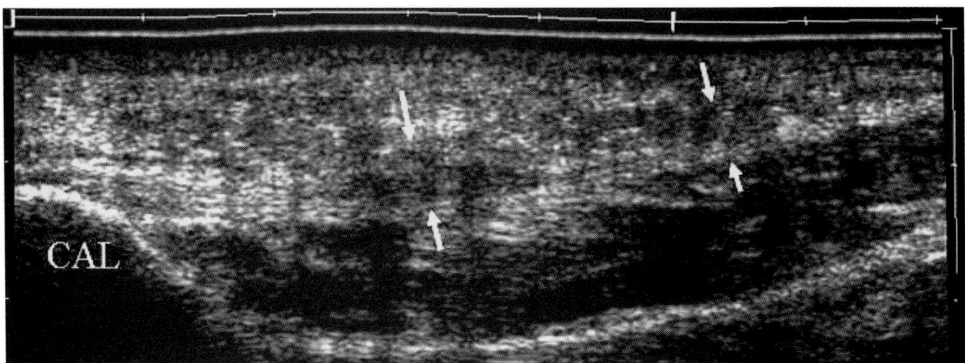

FIG. 5-24. Longitudinal extended field of view image demonstrating multifocal irregular hypoechoic masses within the plantar fascia (*arrows*) consistent with plantar fibromas. Plantar fibromas are often multiple and bilateral. This, along with the fact that the epicenters of the masses are within the plantar fascia, helps to distinguish plantar fibromas from other masses about the foot and ankle, such as synovial sarcomas.

REFERENCES

1. Patel S, Fessell DP, Jacobson JA, et al. Artifacts, anatomic variants and pitfalls in sonography of the foot and ankle. *AJR Am J Roentgenol* 2002;178:1247–1254.
2. Fornage BD. Achilles tendon: ultrasound examination. *Radiology* 1986;159:759–764.
3. Fessell DP, Vanderscheueren GM, Jacobson JA, et al. Ultrasound of the ankle: technique, anatomy, and diagnosis of pathologic conditions. *Radiographics* 1998:18:325–340.
4. Nazarian LN, Rawool NM, Martin CE, et al. Synovial fluid in the hindfoot and ankle: detection of amount and distribution with ultrasound. *Radiology* 1995;197:275–278.
5. Fessell DP, van Holsbeeck MT. Foot and ankle sonography. *Radiol Clin North Am* 1999;37(4):831–858.
6. Sofka CM, Adler RS. Ultrasound guided interventions in the foot and ankle. *Semin Musculoskel Radiol* 2002;6(2):163–168.
7. Cardinal E, Chhem RK, Beauregard CG, et al. Plantar fasciitis: sonographic evaluation. *Radiology* 1996;201: 257–259.
8. Bedi DG, Davidson DM. Plantar fibromatosis: most common sonographic appearance and variations. *J Clin Ultrasound* 2001;29(9):499–505.
9. Griffith JF, Wong TYY, Wong SM, et al. Sonography of plantar fibromatosis. *AJR Am J Roentgenol* 2002;179: 1167–1172.
10. Acevedo JI, Beskin JL. Complications of plantar fascia rupture associated with corticosteroid injection. *Foot Ankle Int* 1998;19(2):91–97.

6

Miscellaneous Topics: Masses, Foreign Bodies

Ultrasound is excellent in distinguishing cystic from solid masses. Differentiating among various solid masses presents a greater problem in that they are often hypoechoic without other distinguishing characteristics. Location, relative hardness, vascularity, and clinical onset can be helpful in the differential diagnosis. Some of the more common masses about the foot and ankle include neuromas in the forefoot (Fig. 6-1) and synovial and ganglion cysts (Figs. 6-2 and 6-3). Occasionally, nodular proliferation of the plantar fascia can result in an aggressive-appearing hypoechoic mass (plantar fibromatosis) (Fig. 6-4). The masses can occur as solitary nodules or can be infiltrative and fusiform (see Chapter 5). They must be distinguished from other neoplasms such as synovial sarcoma (Fig. 6-5) and dermatosarcoma protuberans. Plantar fibromatosis can be multiple and bilateral, favoring the diagnosis over malignancy (1). Other nodular proliferative masses that can mimic soft tissue neoplasms include pigmented villonodular synovitis and giant cell tumor of tendon sheath, both of which may occur in the ankle (Fig. 6-6). Occasionally, foreign body granulomas may appear masslike (Fig. 6-7). Benign neural tumors likewise may present in the ankle (Fig. 6-8), and these may be mistaken for other lesions based on their clinical presentation. Fibrolipomas are well encapsulated and soft, often appearing echogenic (Fig. 6-9).

Sonography has proved to be a useful adjunct to clinical examination in evaluating for retained foreign bodies (2–4). The retained foreign body is usually seen as an echogenic focus, often surrounded by a hypoechoic halo of inflammatory granulation tissue (5) (Figs. 6-10 and 6-11). The presence of the hypoechoic halo aids in the identification of small foreign bodies, especially when embedded in relatively echogenic tissues such as tendons and subcutaneous fat. A palpable mass may develop at the entry point of a foreign body, corresponding to a foreign body granuloma (Fig. 6-7). The real time nature of ultrasound can be used to determine whether a mass is soft or hard, as well as providing guidance for biopsy (Fig. 6-5). Power Doppler can assess whether one is dealing with a vascular or avascular lesion, which may provide information regarding the nature of the mass (Figs. 6-12 and 6-13).

(Text continues on page 104)

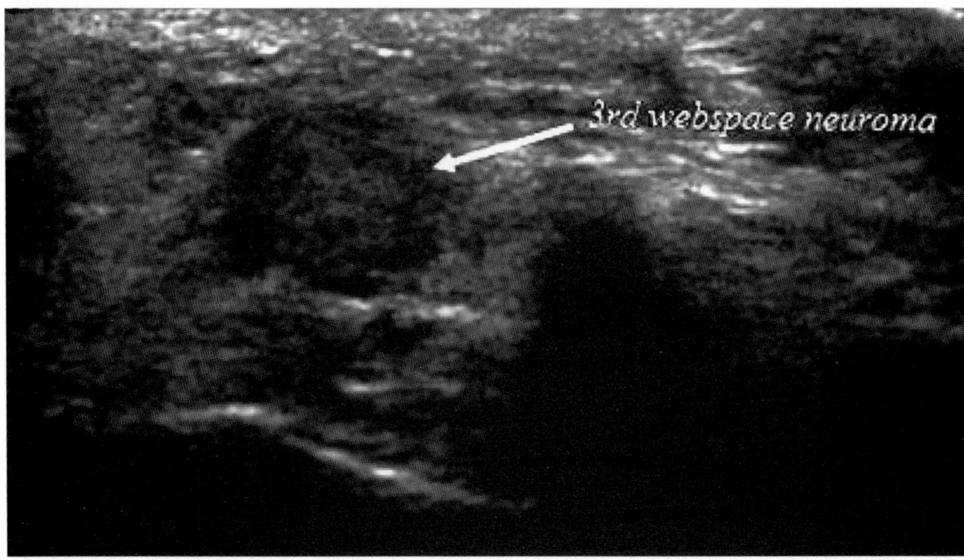

FIG. 6-1. Longitudinal image obtained over the plantar aspect of the third web space demonstrates a discrete hypoechoic nodule that was incompressible. The appearance and location are typical for a Morton neuroma (see Chapter 2).

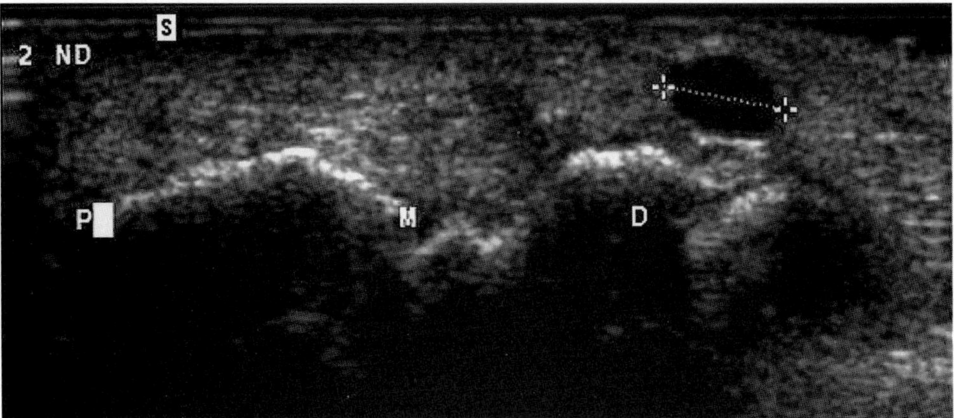

FIG. 6-2. Longitudinal ultrasound image obtained over the plantar aspect of the second toe in a patient with a palpable nodule. A small anechoic mass is present, which is contiguous with the joint capsule of the distal interphalangeal (DIP) joint. Subtle increased sound transmission may be appreciated below the deep margin of the mass. The features are typical for a ganglion cyst. Note that P, M, and D denote proximal, middle and distal phalanges, respectively.

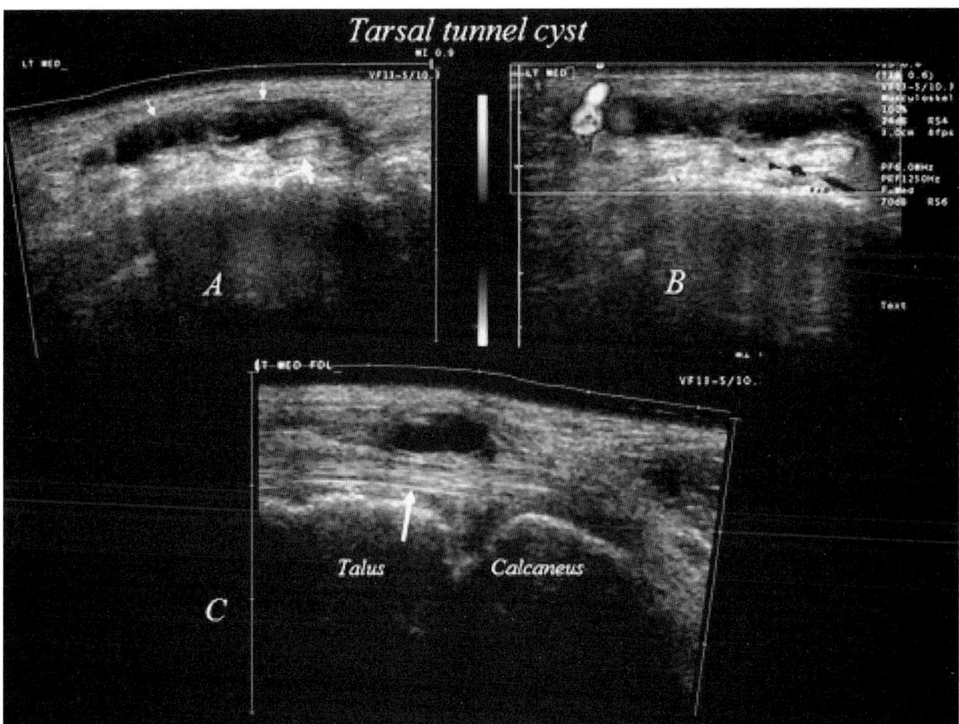

FIG. 6-3. Ganglion cysts are among the most common masses in the foot and ankle. They are hard owing to the nature of the gelatinous material they contain and may compress neurovascular structures. This is particularly evident in the case of tarsal tunnel cysts (depicted here), which can produce posterior tibial nerve compression. **A, B:** Gray scale and power Doppler images of the tarsal tunnel in a patient with paresthesias of the forefoot. A multiloculated ganglion cyst (small arrows) overlies the flexor digitorum longus tendon (big arrow, image A). The relationship to the neurovascular structures is evident when power Doppler is applied. The nerve is poorly visualized here owing to compression by the cyst and overlying vessels. **C:** Long axis image showing a portion of the cyst overlying the flexor digitorum longus tendon (arrow). The talus and calcaneus are labeled.

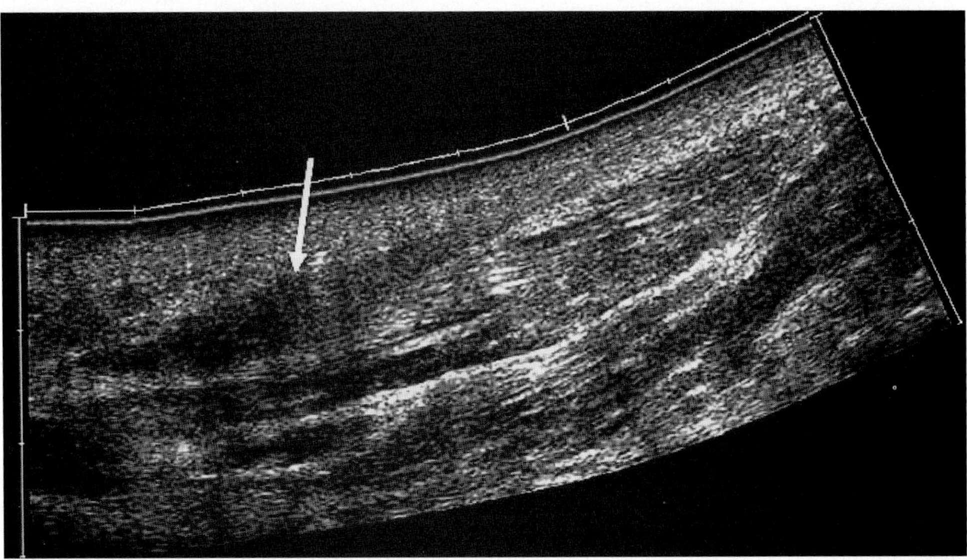

FIG. 6-4. Extended field of view image in a patient with a hard nodular hypoechoic mass (*arrow*) arising from the superficial margin of the plantar fascia. The appearances are in keeping with a large plantar fibroma. On ultrasound, these can appear fairly extensive and aggressive. However, they are always confined to the plantar fascia, helping to differentiate them from more aggressive masses (see Chapter 5).

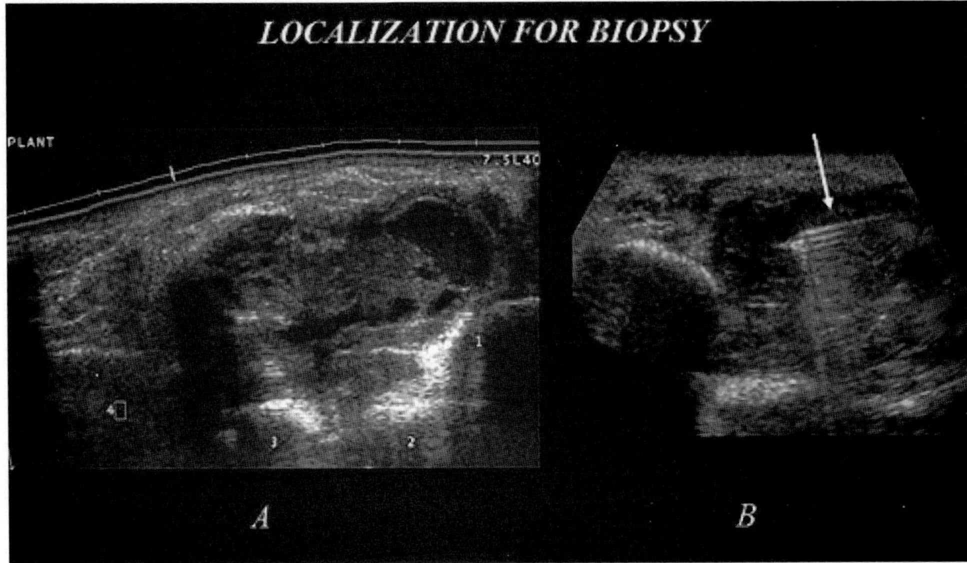

FIG. 6-5. A: Extended field of view transverse image in a patient who had a history of a Morton neuroma resection 1 year earlier. The metatarsals, seen in cross section, are labeled. A large hypoechoic mass containing cystic spaces is present. On power Doppler (not shown), the mass was hypervascular. **B:** Transverse view of the plantar aspect of the foot during ultrasound-guided biopsy. The needle was directed to a solid portion of the tumor, and multiple core biopsy samples were obtained. Synovial cell sarcoma was diagnosed.

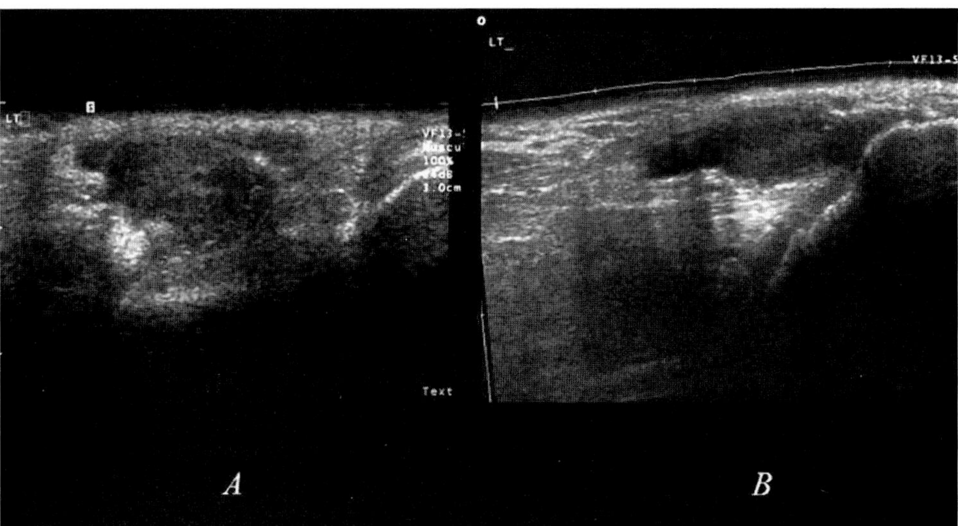

FIG. 6-6. Transverse **(A)** and longitudinal **(B)** images of the tarsal tunnel in a patient with a palpable mass. An irregular hypoechoic mass is seen contiguous with the flexor hallucis longus tendon. **A:** The tendon appears as an echogenic circular structure along the inferior left margin of the mass. **B:** The mass is well defined and situated along the superficial margin of the tendon. The mass demonstrated moderate vascularity on power Doppler imaging (not shown), without cystic components. The ultrasound appearance of the mass is not specific. In this case, a giant cell tumor of tendon sheath was diagnosed, although a soft tissue sarcoma could also present a similar appearance. Further characterization of the mass with magnetic resonance imaging and biopsy would be required for further evaluation.

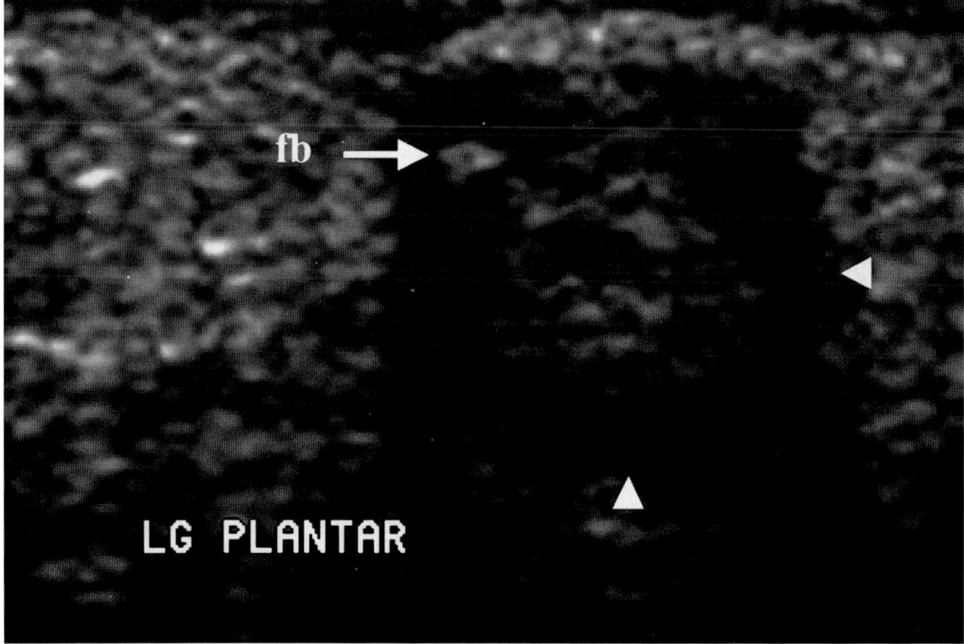

FIG. 6-7. Longitudinal ultrasound image obtained at the site of a palpable nodule along the plantar aspect of the foot. The patient gave a history of a remote puncture injury to the foot while walking on the beach and of removing shell fragments from the wound. A discrete heterogeneous nodule (*arrowheads*) is present with a hypoechoic halo. A small echogenic area within the periphery of the nodule was shown to correspond to a small residual shell fragment. In this case, a foreign-body granuloma was diagnosed, which presented clinically as a painful hard mass.

A

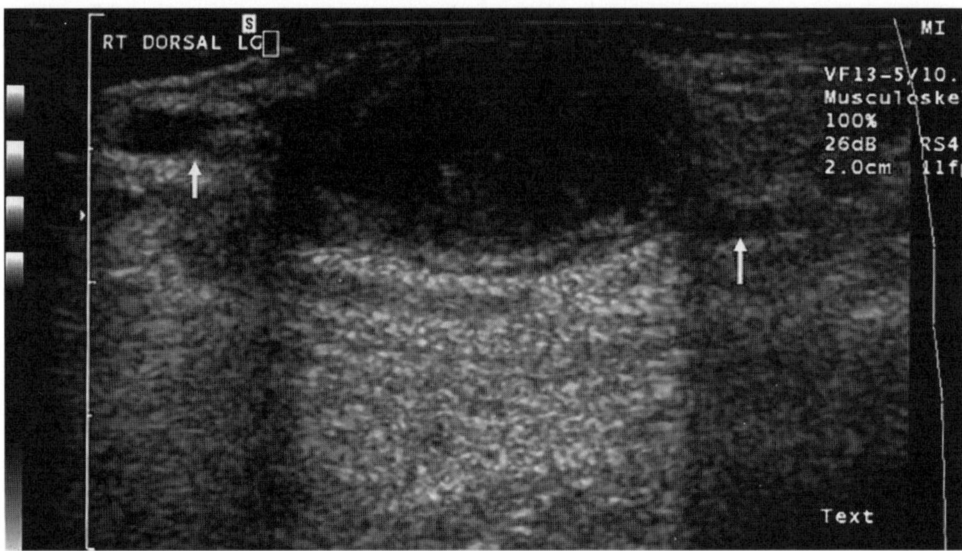

B

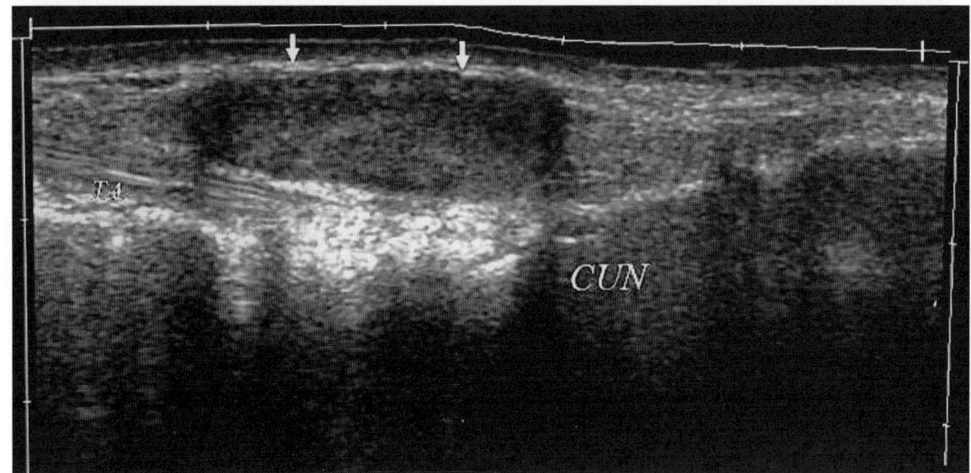

FIG. 6-8. A: The relationship of masses to regional neurovascular structures can be defined with sonography. This longitudinal image demonstrates a well-defined hypoechoic mass within the substance of the deep peroneal nerve (the more normal proximal and distal aspects of the nerve can be seen (*arrows*) consistent with a neurofibroma. The presence of a nerve having entry and exit points relative to such a mass is pathognomonic for a neural tumor. **B:** The presence of a nerve in relation to a neural tumor is not always evident. Longitudinal extended field of view image of the dorsum of the midfoot demonstrates a well-defined hypoechoic mass consistent with a neurofibroma (*arrows*). Note the proximity of the mass to the medial cuneiform (CUN) and the tibialis anterior tendon (TA).

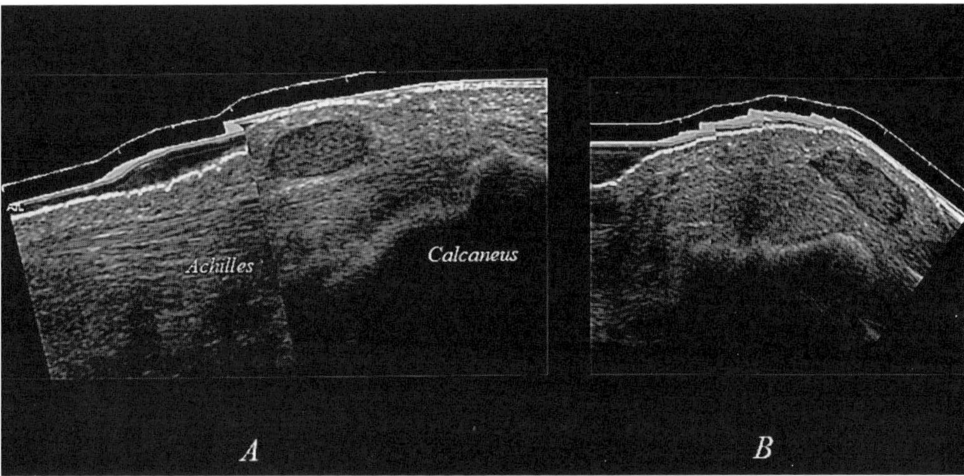

FIG. 6-9. Longitudinal **(A)** and transverse **(B)** extended field of view images of a soft palpable nodule along the lateral margin of the posterior ankle. An echogenic mass, which is encapsulated, is present in the subcutaneous fat along the lateral margin of the Achilles tendon. The mass is slightly less echogenic than the adjacent fat. The appearances are in keeping with a fibrolipoma. Most fatty tumors are isoechoic or hyperechoic relative to the adjacent fat. Enthesopathic changes are incidentally noted at the tendon insertion onto the calcaneus.

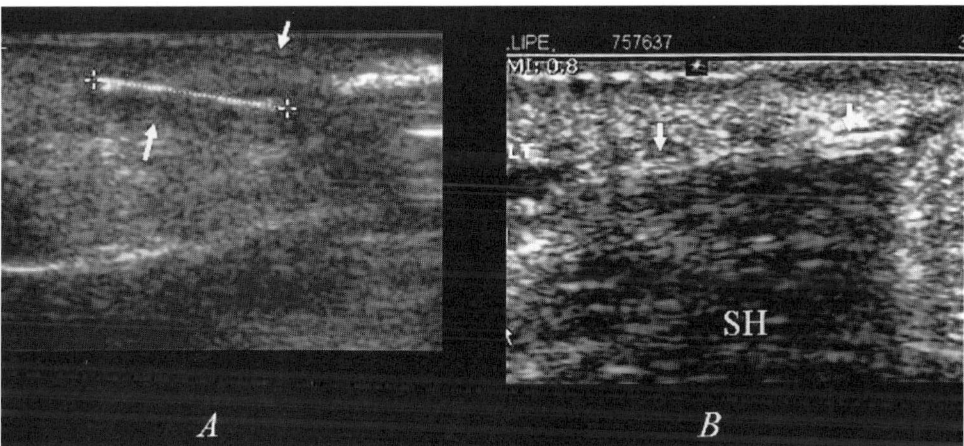

FIG. 6-10. Foreign bodies typically appear as linear strong reflectors. **A:** As a result of the inflammatory response of the adjacent soft tissue, a surrounding hypoechoic halo may be present, increasing their conspicuity on ultrasound. **B:** Foreign bodies may also display a clean or dirty shadow (SH), as in the second example presented.

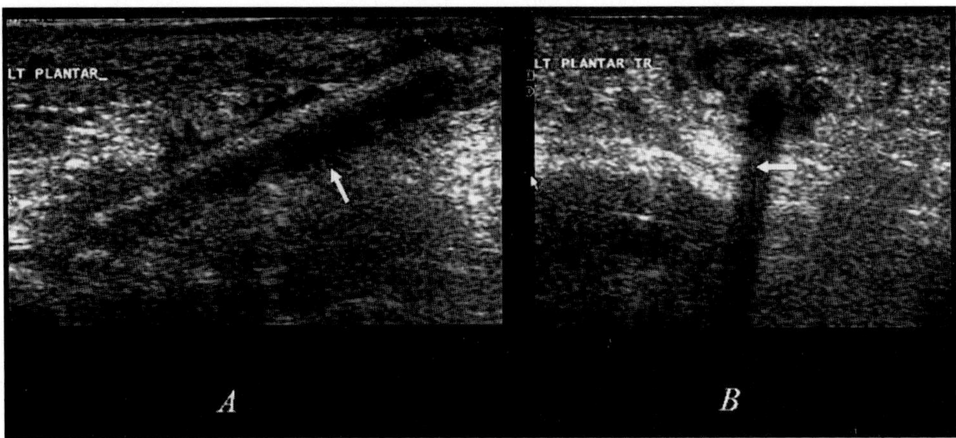

FIG. 6-11. Longitudinal **(A)** and transverse **(B)** images of the foot in a patient who had stepped on a cocktail toothpick. Clinical concern was of a retained foreign body. Identification of foreign bodies is often aided by identifying a hypoechoic rim around the foreign body (**A**, *arrow*). Occasionally, foreign bodies demonstrate posterior acoustic shadowing (**B**, *arrow*).

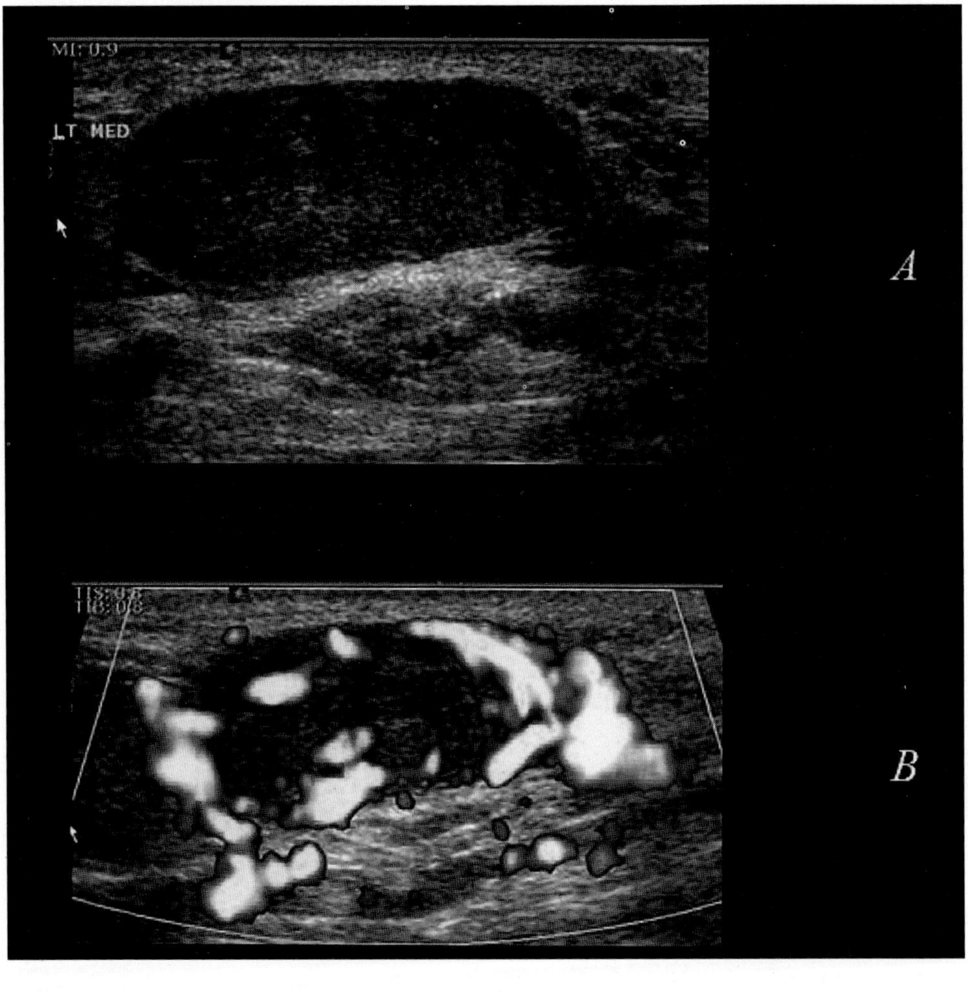

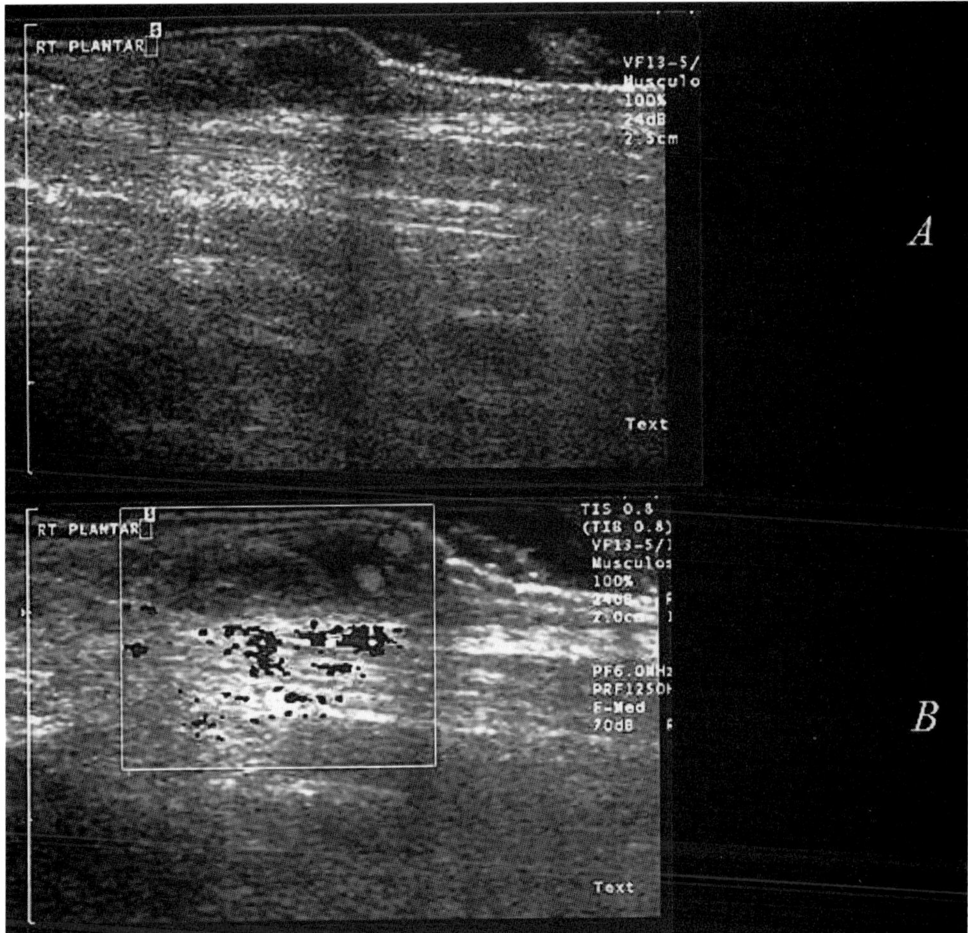

FIG. 6-13. A: Longitudinal image of the plantar aspect of the midfoot demonstrates a subcutaneous heterogeneous mass in the plantar aspect of the foot. **B:** Application of Power Doppler demonstrates some prominent internal veins, consistent with a small vascular malformation, most likely a cavernous hemangioma.

FIG. 6-12. A: Longitudinal gray scale image along the plantar medial aspect of the ankle demonstrates a well-defined hypoechoic mass that was soft to palpation with the transducer. **B:** The application of power Doppler confirms that this is a vascular lesion. Spectral Doppler analysis (not shown) demonstrates multiple enlarged arteries and veins with arterialized venous flow. The sonographic appearance is characteristic of an arteriovenous malformation.

REFERENCES

1. Griffith JF, Wong TY, Wong SM, et al. Sonography of plantar fibromatosis. *AJR Am J Roentgenol* 2002;179 (5):1167–1172.
2. Jacobson JA, Powell A, Craig JG, et al. *Radiology* 1998;206(1):45–48.
3. Rockett MS, Gentile SC, Gudas CJ, et al. The use of ultrasonography for the detection of retained wooden foreign bodies in the foot. *J Foot Ankle Surg* 1995;34(5):478–484.
4. Peterson JJ, Bancroft LW, Kransdorf MJ. Wooden foreign bodies: imaging appearance. *AJR Am J Roentgenol* 2002;178(3):557–562.
5. Fornage BD, Schernberg FJ. Sonographic diagnosis of foreign bodies of the distal extremities. *AJR Am J Roentgenol* 1986:147;567–569.

7

Percutaneous Ultrasound-Guided Procedures in the Foot and Ankle

Ultrasound guidance for percutaneous procedures has been employed for years in the vascular system as well as for various visceral interventions such as liver, thyroid, and breast biopsies. Several reports have demonstrated the utility of sonographic guidance for percutaneous procedures in the musculoskeletal system, including joint aspirations and ganglion cyst aspirations and injections (1–6).

The superficial nature of the structures within the foot and ankle make them amenable to sonographically guided interventions. Structures that can be targeted for ultrasound-guided interventions in the foot and ankle include ganglion and synovial cysts (see Chapter 3), joints (Figs. 7-1 and 7-2), tendon sheaths (Figs. 7-3 and 7-4), Morton's neuromas (Fig. 7-5), plantar fascia (Fig. 7-6), and bursae (Fig. 7-7). Likewise, aspirations or biopsies can be performed (Fig. 7-8; see also Chapter 6). Although somewhat unusual in the ankle, ultrasound-guided calcium fragmentation and aspiration has been shown to be effective in other locations within the musculoskeletal system (Fig. 7-9).

The echogenic needle often demonstrates a characteristic posterior reverberation artifact (Fig. 7-7). Advantages of ultrasound-guided percutaneous interventions over blind injections include the ability to visualize adjacent structures, such as neurovascular bundles, directly and thus to avoid them, as well as the ability to identify the needle tip clearly within the target of interest (Fig. 7-10). This is especially useful in terms of joint aspirations. If the tibiotalar joint is aspirated blindly, for example, and there is a dry tap, the clinician is uncertain whether there truly was no fluid in the joint or he or she missed the target. With direct ultrasound visualization, one can clearly see the needle tip within the hypoechoic joint space, thus resulting in accurate deposition of therapeutic agent (Figs. 7-1 and 7-2).

In general, for foot and ankle injections, either a high- or medium-frequency linear transducer is employed. The area of interest should be cleaned and draped in a sterile manner, using an iodine-based solution if there are no contraindications such as allergy to topical iodine (Fig. 7-11). Either a longitudinal or short axis approach can be employed (Figs. 7-12 and 7-13); however, a short axis approach is often technically easier for tendon sheath, bursal, and small joint injections to avoid intratendinous injections (2) (Figs. 7-13 to 7–15). The needle should enter the skin, paralleling the long axis of the transducer (Figs. 7-5 to 7–7). Ideally, the needle should be in direct view at all times. At our institution, we typically employ 1% lidocaine for local anesthesia and inject from 0.5 to 2 mL of a steroid-anesthetic mixture, depending on the distensibility and size of the region of interest. Typically, a mixture composed of ¼ 1% lidocaine, ¼ 0.5% bupivacaine, and ½ triamcinolone is used.

(Text continues on page 118)

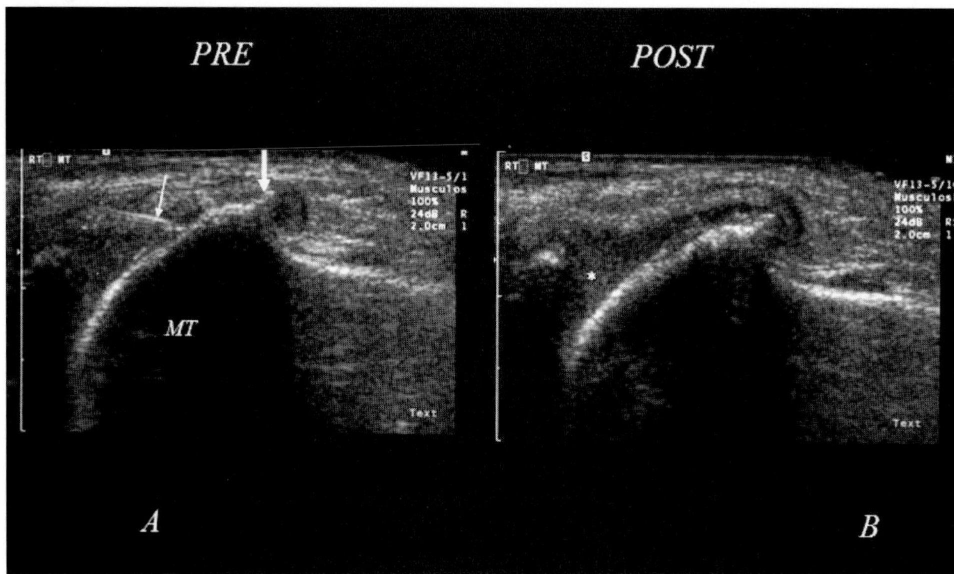

FIG. 7-1. The metatarsophalangeal (MTP) joints of the forefoot can be injected from a longitudinal approach (along the axis of the joint) as well as a short axis approach (in the plane parallel to the joint). **A:** Longitudinal ultrasound image of the first MTP joint for injection. The first metatarsal head (MT) demonstrates a large dorsal osteophyte from osteoarthritis (*short thick white arrow*). Linear echogenic needle tip is seen within the joint space (*short thin white arrow*). There is some hypoechoic debris distending the joint space, consistent with inflammatory synovitis. **B:** Subsequent image on the right obtained after injection demonstrates fluid containing multiple low-level echoes now distending the joint space (*asterisk*). It should be noted that the therapeutic mixture itself contributes to low-level echoes within the distended joint capsule.

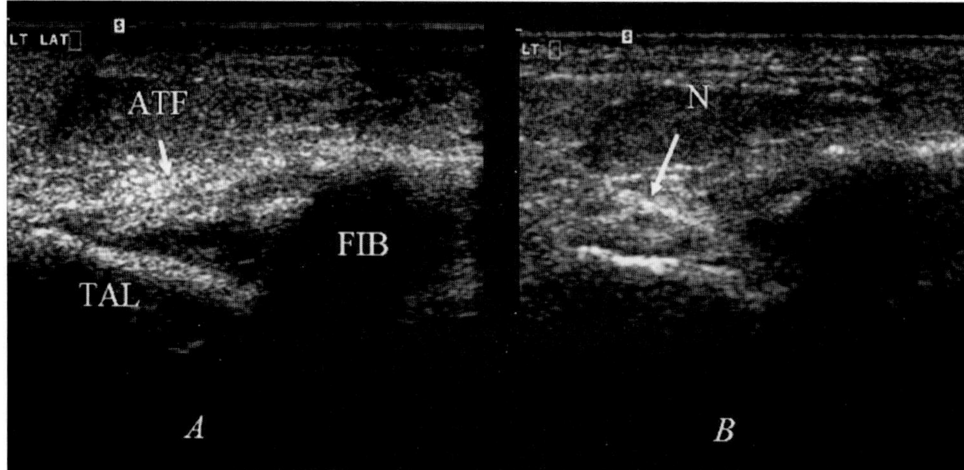

FIG. 7-2. Injection of the lateral gutter may be performed as a simple method to approach the tibiotalar joint or in cases of anterolateral impingement. We employ a 1.5-inch 25-gauge needle and a short axis approach. **A:** Direct imaging over the anterior talofibular ligament (ATF) displays the exposed portion of the lateral gutter, which contains hypoechoic fluid and debris. **B:** An echogenic needle (N) is seen within the gutter. Numerous echoes within this space correspond to the therapeutic mixture injected.

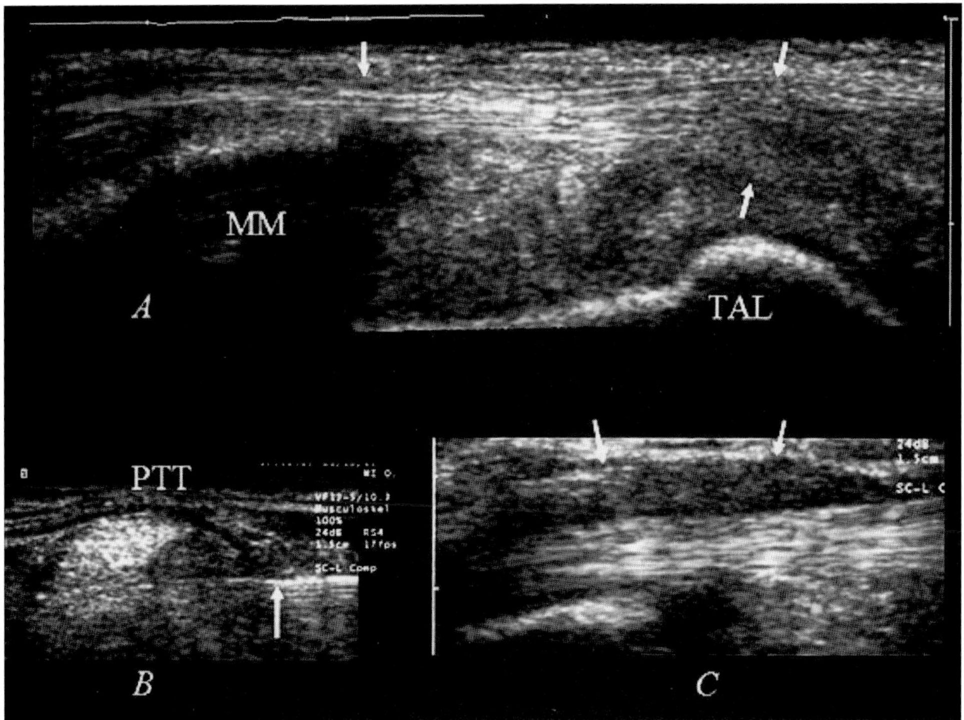

FIG. 7-3. Various tendon sheaths about the foot and ankle can be injected. **A:** This is a longitudinal image demonstrating moderate distal posterior tibial tendinosis (*short arrows*). The medial malleolus (MM) and talus (TAL) are labeled. **B:** A needle was placed within the deep margin of the posterior tendon (PTT) sheath from a short axis approach (*arrow*). **C:** Hypoechoic material can be seen distending the tendon sheath (*long axis view*) after the injection and needle removal (*arrows*). The steroid-anesthetic mixture typically contains low-level echoes.

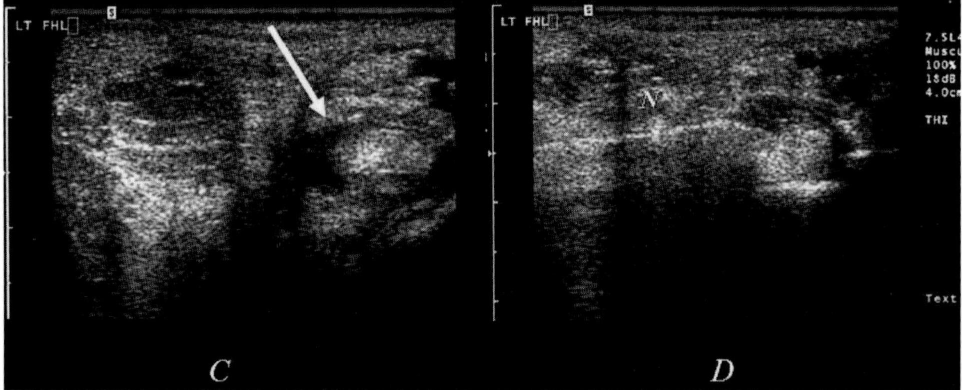

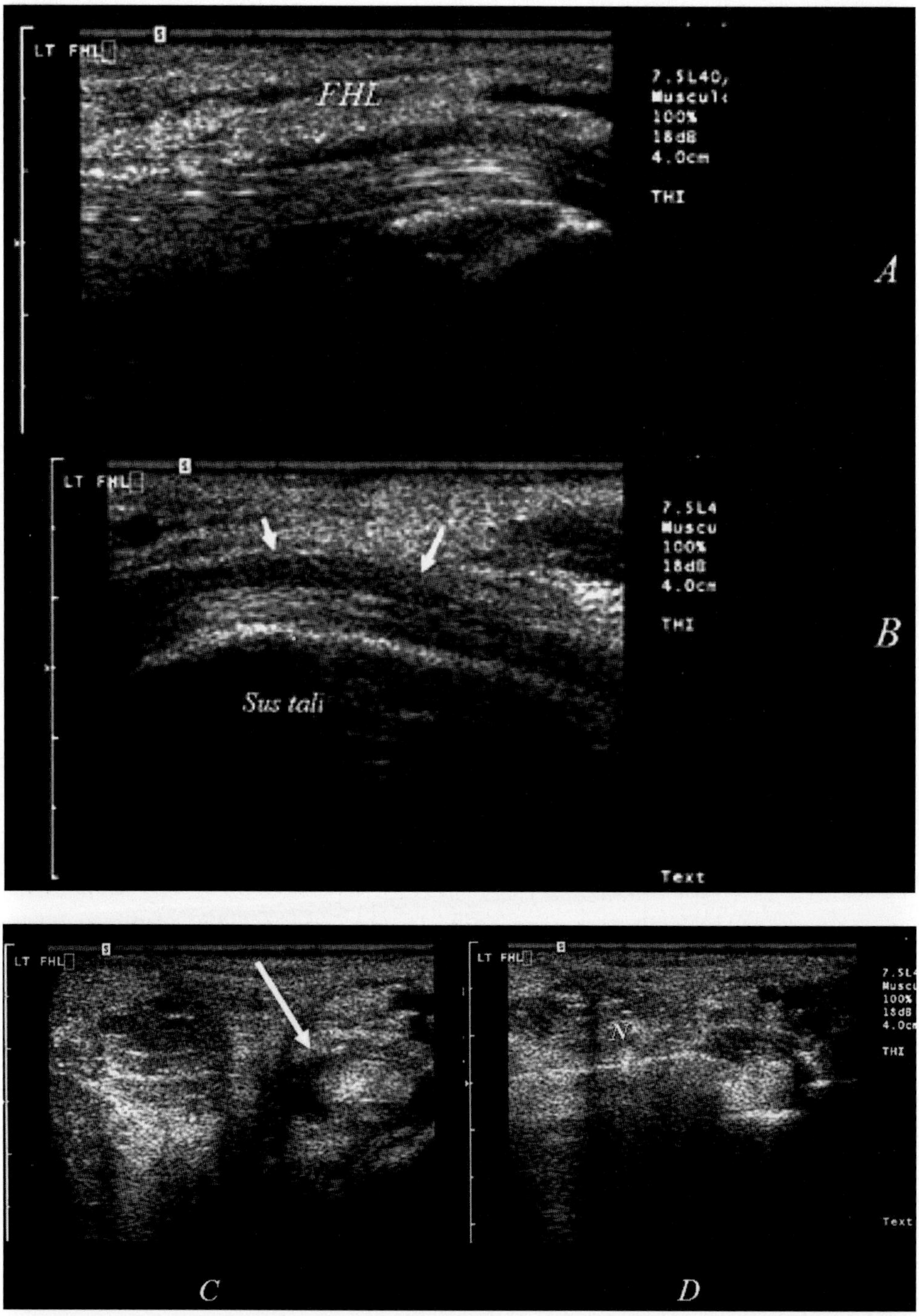

FIG. 7-4. Longitudinal images of the flexor hallucis longus tendon (FHL) proximal to **(A)** and below **(B)** the sustentaculum tali (sus tal). These images demonstrate moderate tendon sheath thickening (*arrows*). **C:** Short axis view of the FHL at the level of the posterior talus. Moderate eccentric thickening of the tendon sheath is evident (*arrow*). **D:** A needle was inserted into the tendon sheath from a short axis approach, and hypoechoic material can be seen distending the tendon sheath.

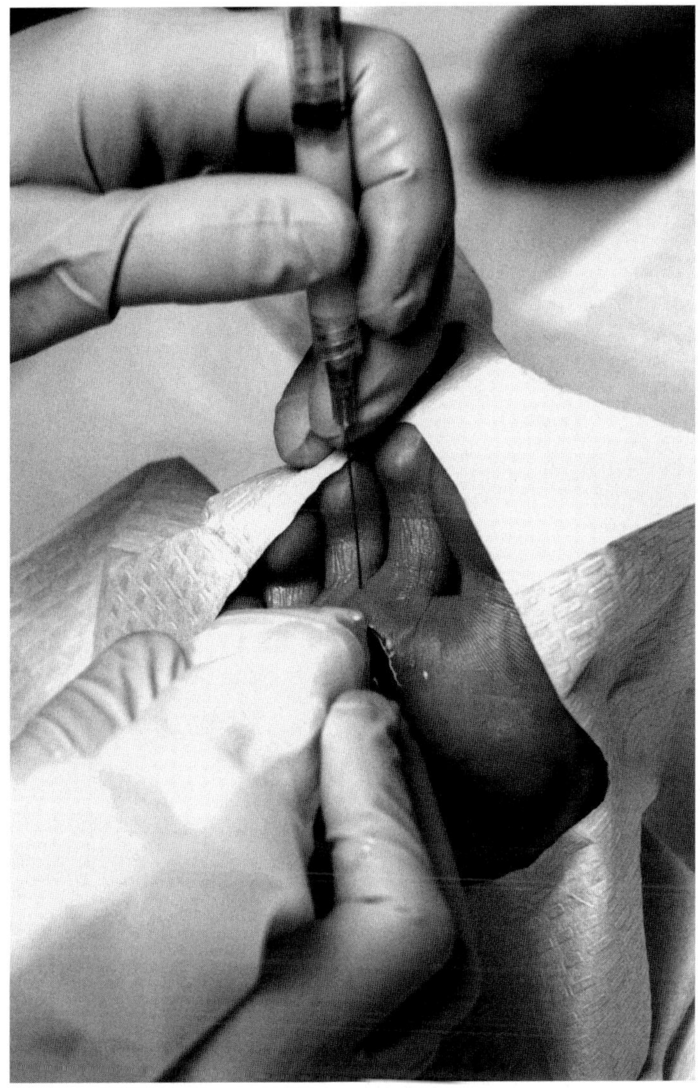

A

FIG. 7-5. A: Intermetatarsal neuromas can be injected from either a dorsal or a plantar approach. For the plantar approach, the foot is dorsiflexed, and the web space is addressed from the plantar margin.

FIG. 7-5. *(Continued on next page)*

B

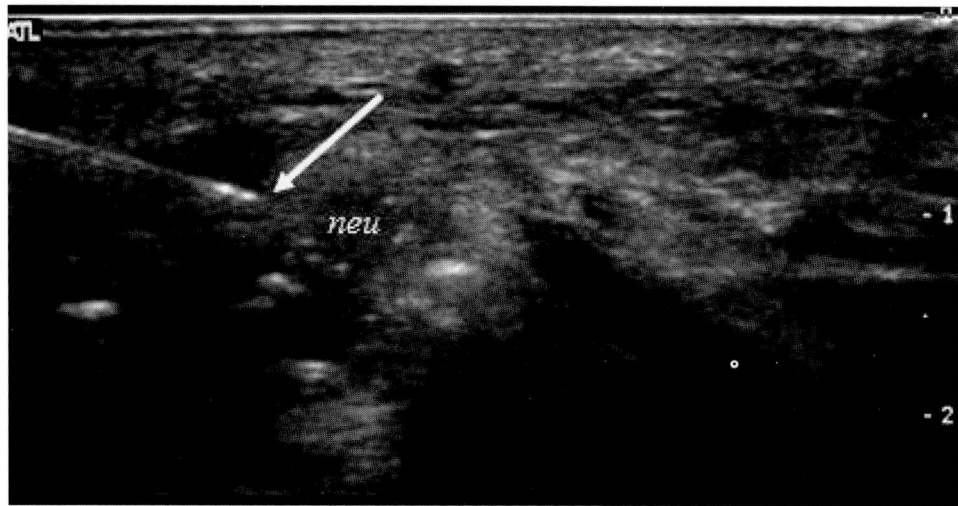

C

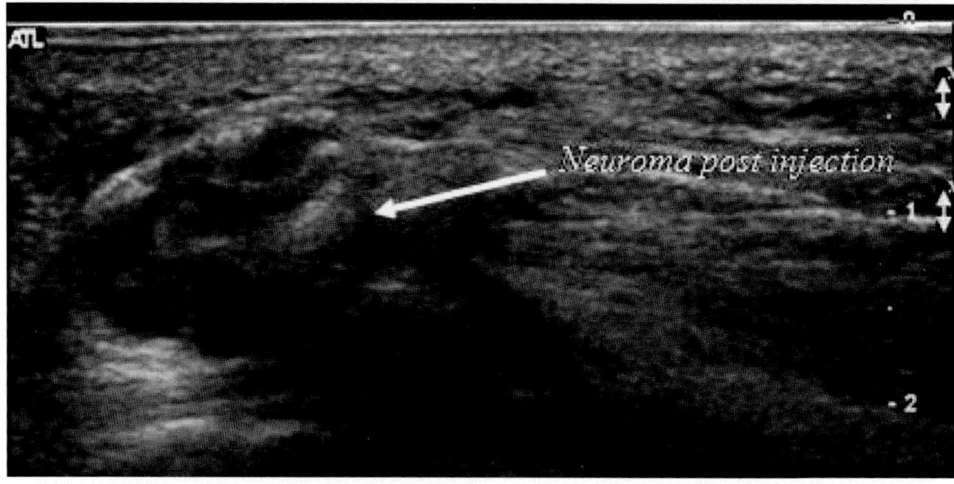

FIG. 7-5. B: Longitudinal image demonstrating a needle tip (*arrow*) within a large hypoechoic neuroma (neu). **C:** After removal of the needle, the neuroma demonstrates increased internal echoes. In some instances, an associated intermetatarsal bursa fills.

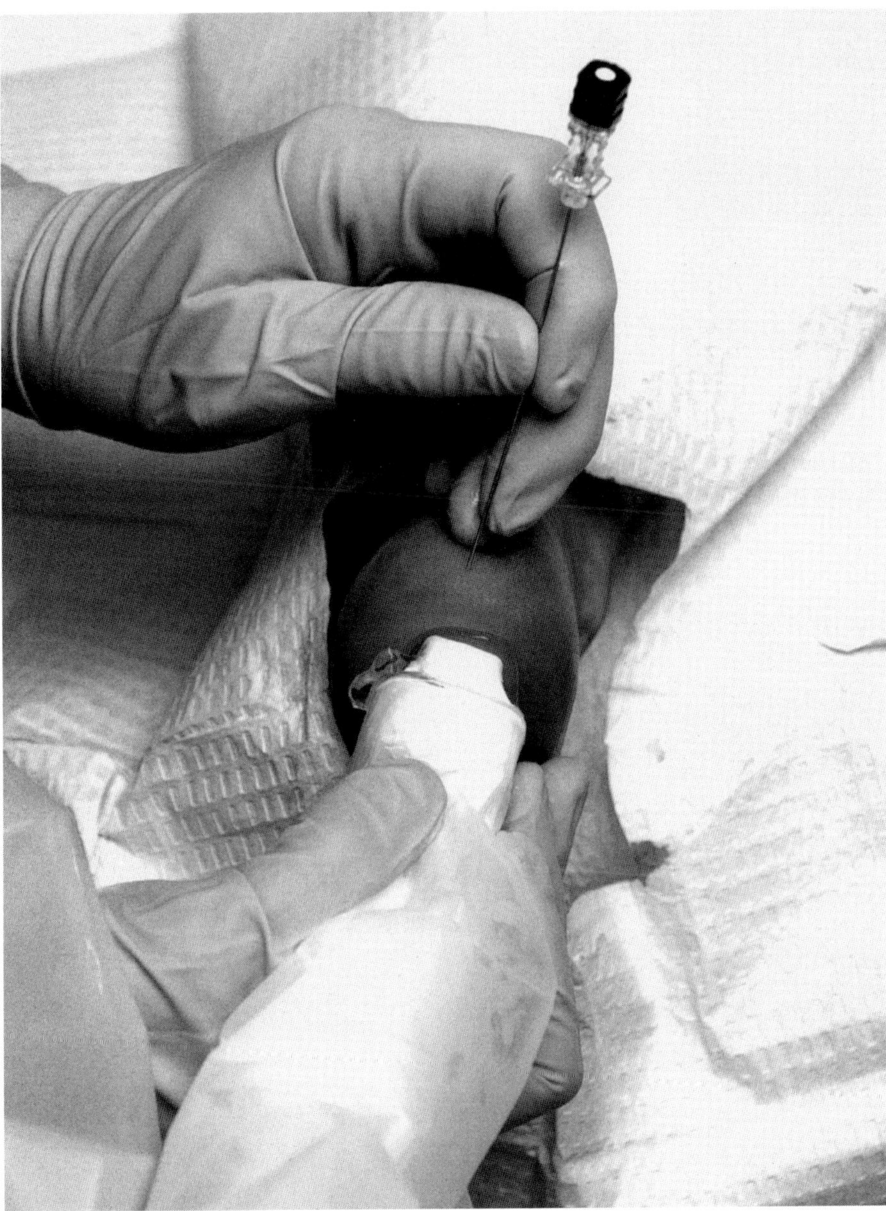

FIG. 7-6. Typical setup for injection of the plantar fascia. The patient is prone and the foot dorsiflexed. Typically, the plantar fascia is injected from a longitudinal approach. A spinal needle is typically used because the skin over the heel can be moderately thick. The spinal needle is directed longitudinally, superficial (plantar) to the plantar fascia, where the steroid-anesthetic mixture is injected.

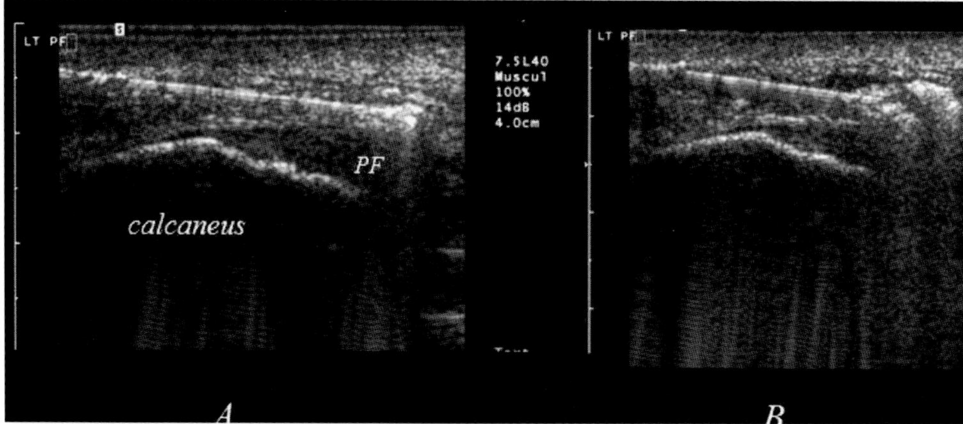

FIG. 7-7. A: Longitudinal ultrasound image of a plantar fascia injection. The calcaneus and plantar fascia (PF) are indicated. A spinal needle is placed within the skin in the heel region and directed toward the superficial medial origin of the plantar fascia, avoiding direct intrafascial injection, which has been associated with plantar fascia rupture. **B:** Subsequent image demonstrates injection of the steroid-anesthetic mixture with multiple low-level echoes seen superficial to the plantar fascia, which typically distributes circumferentially about the superficial margin of the fascia.

A

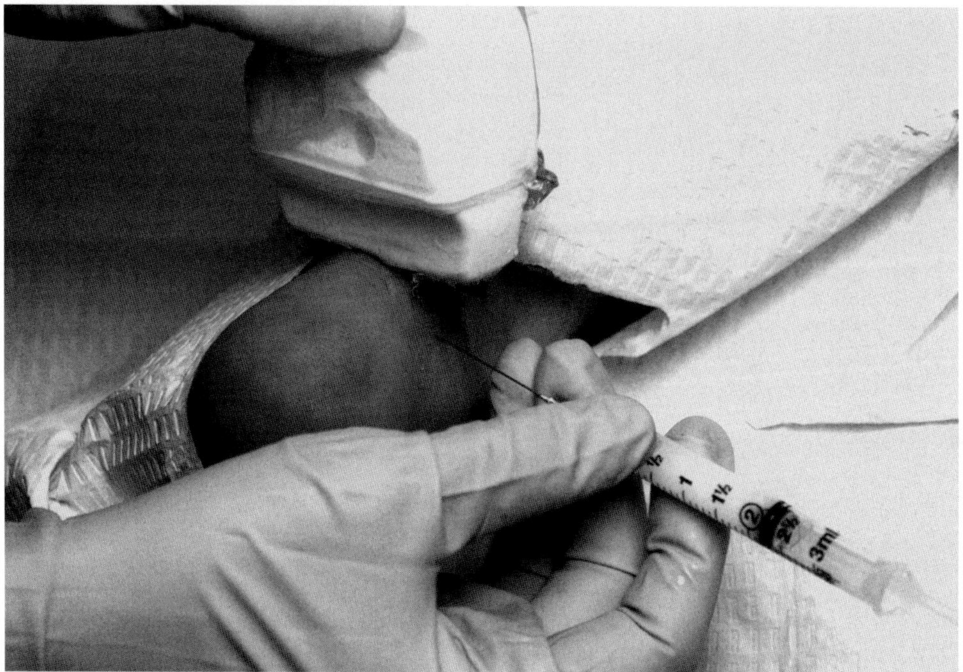

FIG. 7-8. A: A short axis approach is typically used to enter the retrocalcaneal bursa. The transducer is placed over the posterior ankle at the level of the bursa. The needle is positioned to see it optimally as a strong specular reflector.

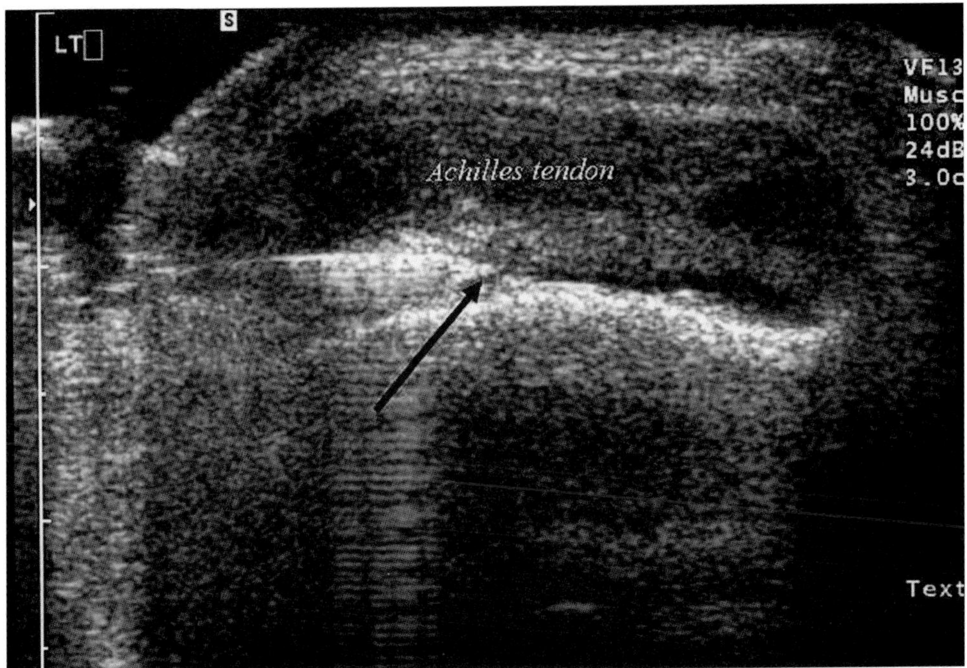

B

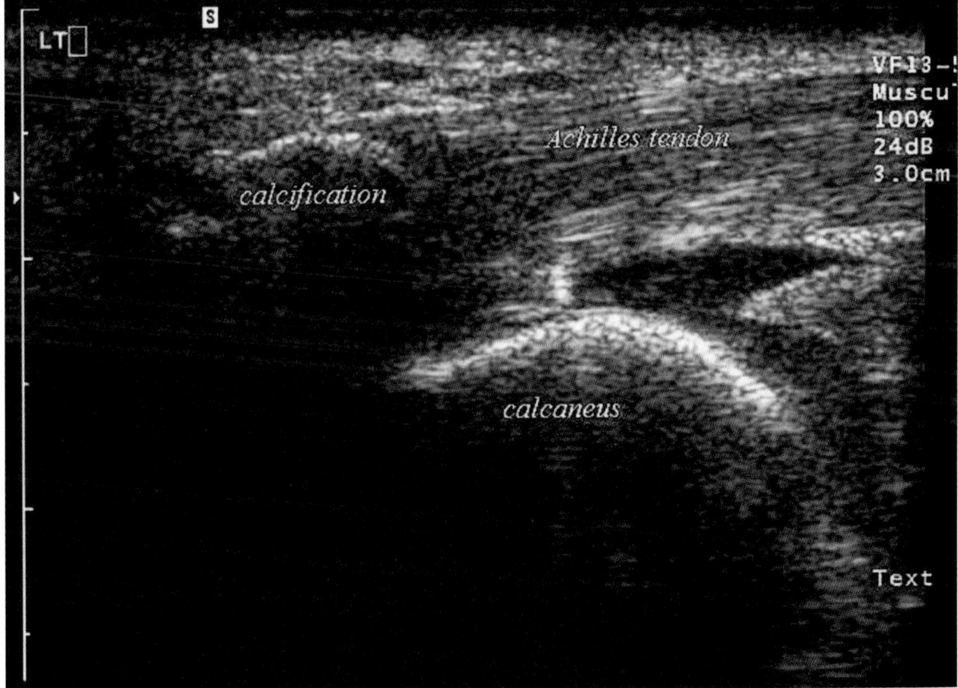

C

FIG. 7-8. B: Axial image demonstrating a needle entering the deep retrocalcaneal bursa from a short axis approach (*arrow*). A strong reverberation artifact can be appreciated deep to the needle. Only a small amount of fluid was present in the bursa before the injection. **C:** On this longitudinal postinjection image of the distal Achilles tendon, the bursa is distended with the steroid-anesthetic mixture, containing low-level echoes. A large enthesophyte is incidentally noted (calcification).

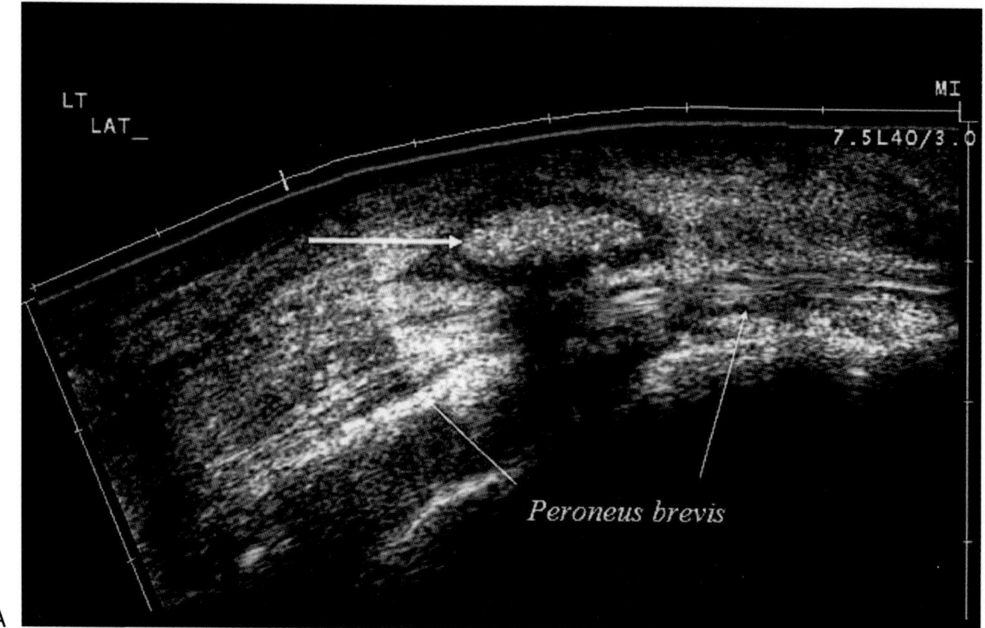

A

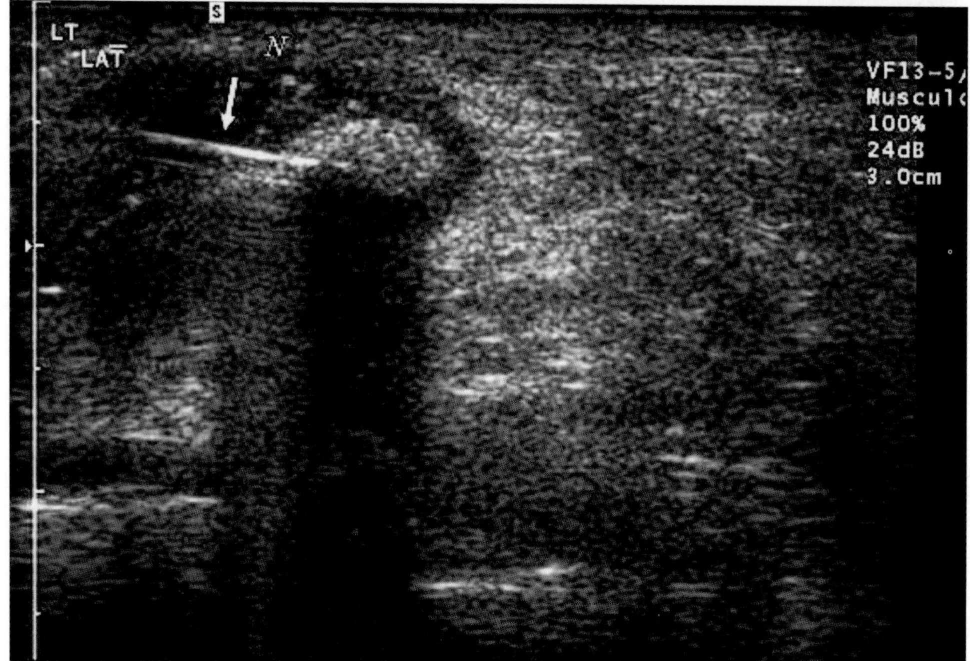

B

FIG. 7-9. A: Longitudinal ultrasound image along the lateral aspect of the ankle in a patient with lateral ankle pain. Preliminary gray scale evaluation demonstrates an oval shadowing echogenic focus within the peroneal tendon sheath, consistent with calcification. **B:** This area was addressed for percutaneous aspiration and mechanical decompression. The echogenic needle tip (N) can be seen within the substance of the calcification.

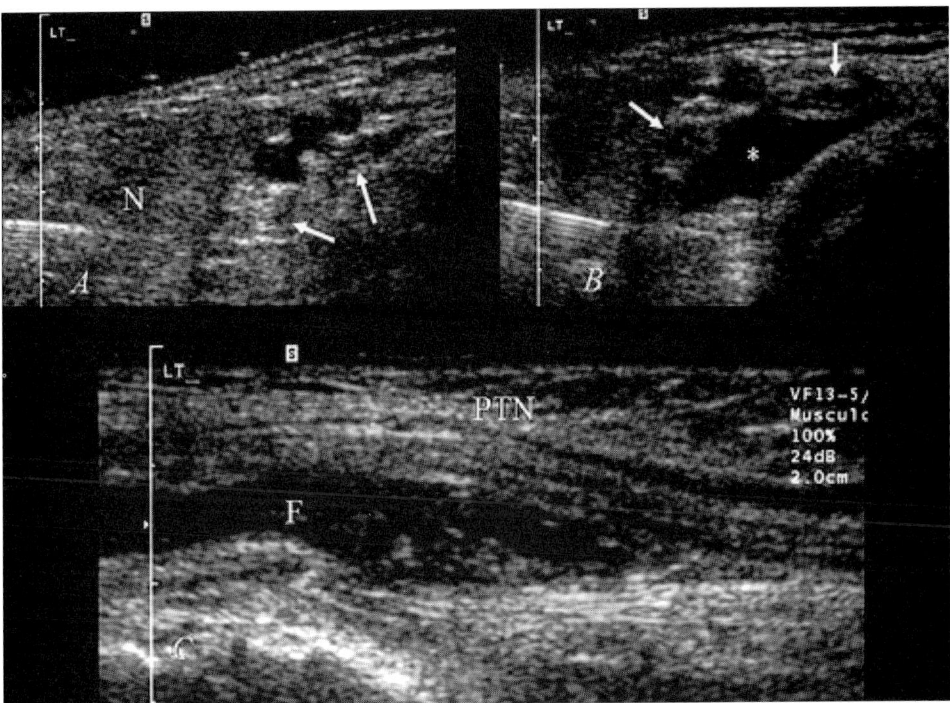

FIG. 7-10. A: Transverse image obtained over the posteromedial ankle during performance of a posterior tibial nerve block. A needle (N) is present below the nerve at the level of its bifurcation into medial and lateral plantar branches. **B:** During the injection of a lidocaine and bupivacaine [Marcaine] mixture, fluid (*asterisk*) fills a space between the needle and the nerve branches. Note that the presence of fluid increases the conspicuity of both the needle and the nerve. **C:** After injection, this longitudinal view of the posterior tibial nerve (PTN) illustrates the distribution of the anesthetic mixture (F) along the course of the nerve, without infiltration of the nerve substance.

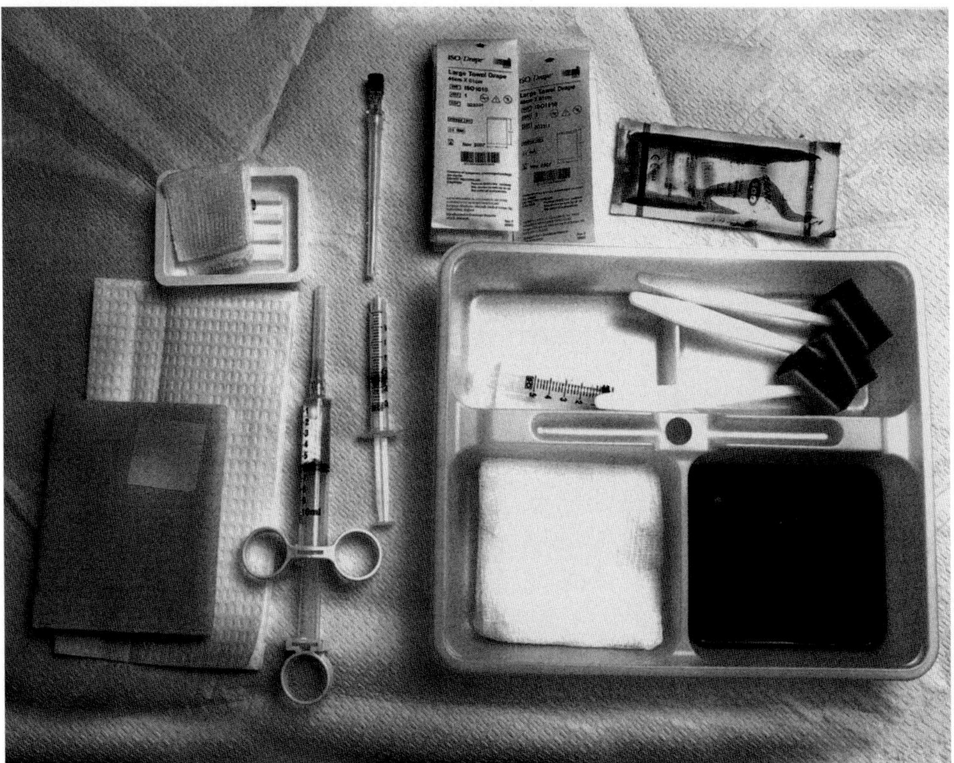

FIG. 7-11. Standard ultrasound-guided procedure setup includes the following items (**clockwise from top left**): an interventional needle (spinal needle can be used for deeper structures: however, in the foot and ankle, a shorter, 1.5-inch needle usually suffices); sterile drapes for the ultrasound probe; sterile ultrasound gel; a custom tray kit with an iodine solution used for cleaning; the steroid mixture to be injected; a syringe with local anesthesia; and various sterile drapes.

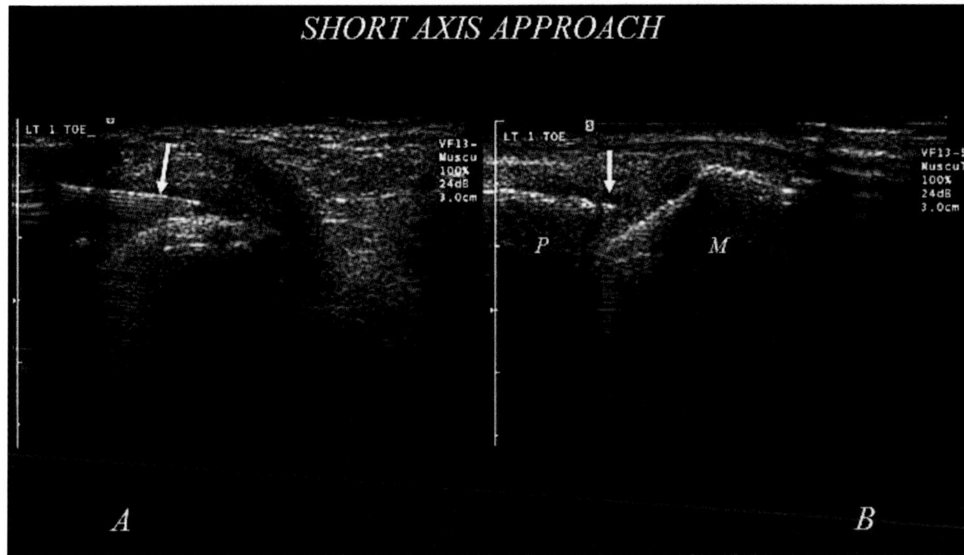

FIG. 7-12. Joints of the forefoot can also be injected from a short axis approach. **A:** In this example, the first metatarsophalangeal (MTP) joint is being addressed for injection from a short axis approach. The skin entry site is typically medial to the first MTP joint, and the needle is placed into the joint, near the first metatarsal head (*arrow*). **B:** The image on the **right** is a longitudinal image demonstrating the metatarsal head (M) as well as the proximal phalanx (P) and the needle tip seen in short axis (*arrow*), with posterior reverberation artifact.

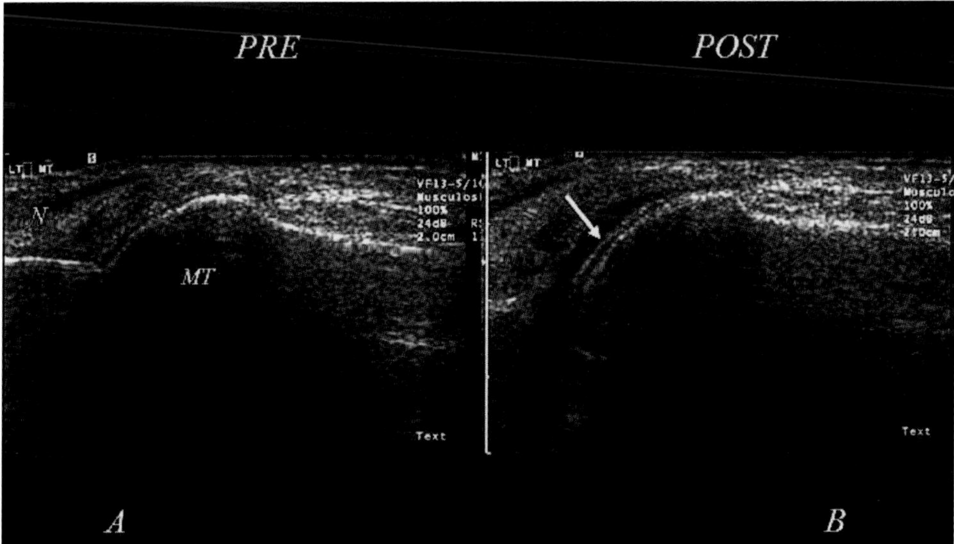

FIG. 7-13. A long axis approach may also be of value at times because the needle can be more readily adjusted during the injection or if the joint is not accessible from a short axis approach. In this case, a first metatarsophalangeal (MTP) joint injection was requested. **A:** A short 25-gauge needle is present (N) with its tip along the articular surface of the first metatarsal head (MT). **B:** After injection and needle removal, there is distention of the dorsal recess by fluid. The articular cartilage (*arrow*) is more readily apparent.

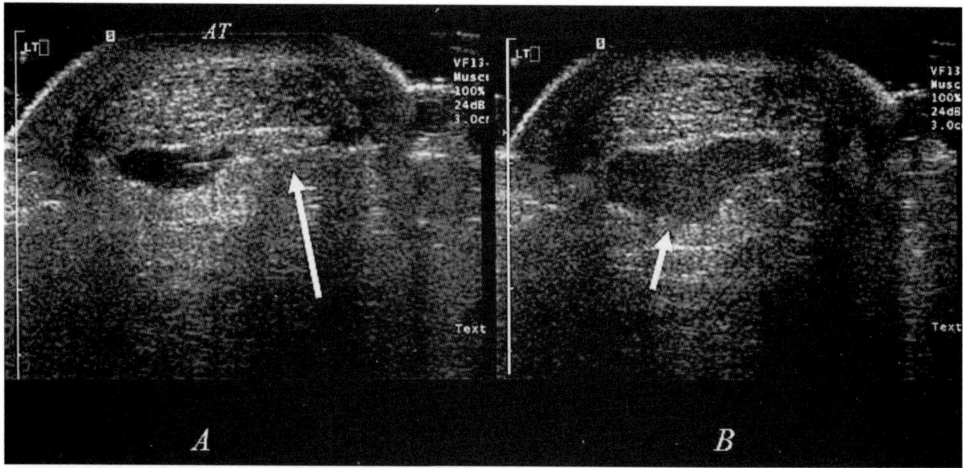

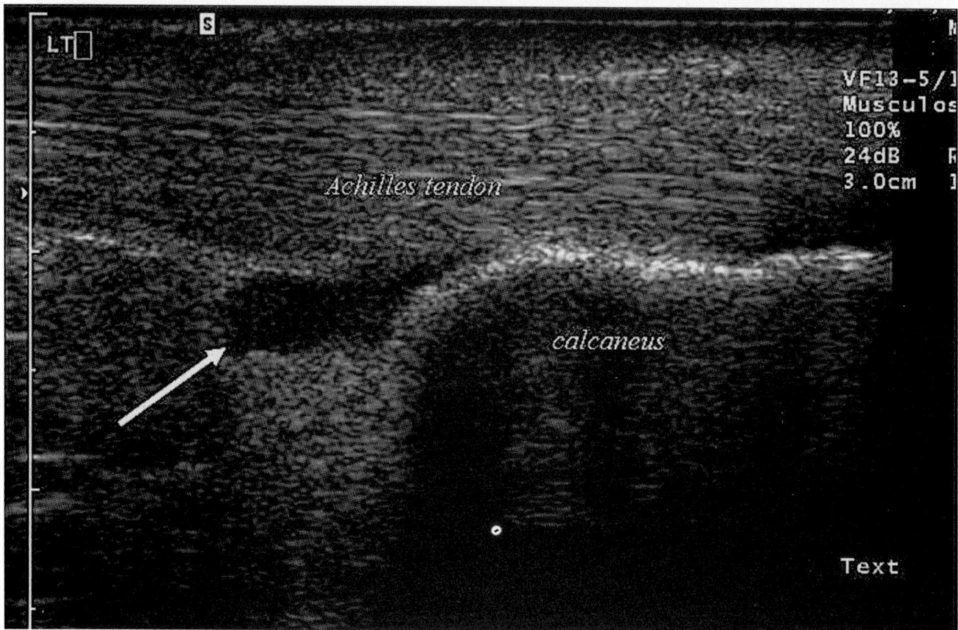

FIG. 7-14. A: Short axis view of the Achilles tendon (AT) demonstrates a needle within the deep retrocalcaneal bursa (*arrow*). **B:** The bursa is now distended (observed in real time) with hypoechoic material corresponding to the steroid-anesthetic mixture. One advantage of ultrasound is the ability to provide continuous real time monitoring of the injection. **C:** Longitudinal image demonstrating the steroid-anesthetic mixture in the deep retrocalcaneal bursa (*arrow*).

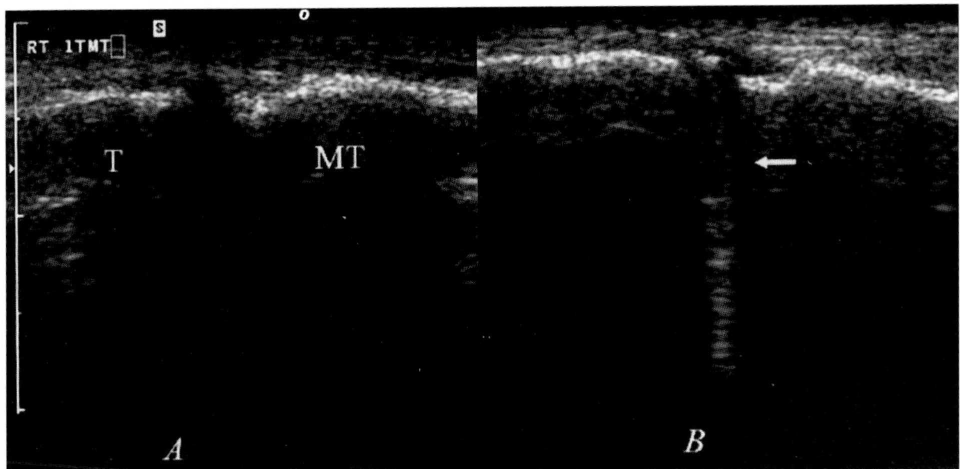

FIG. 7-15. Midfoot injections generally require a short axis approach. In this case, anesthetic alone was injected into the first tarsometatarsal (TMT) joint under ultrasound guidance. **A:** The first TMT joint is imaged in long axis, showing a small joint space without joint fluid or hypertrophic change. **B:** An echogenic needle is present in the joint (seen in short axis). The needle is easily identified as a result of a characteristic ring-down artifact (*arrow*).

REFERENCES

1. Sofka CM, Collins AJ, Adler RS. Use of ultrasonographic guidance in interventional musculoskeletal procedures: a review from a single institution. *J Ultrasound Med* 2001;20:21–26.
2. Adler RS, Sofka CM. Percutaneous ultrasound-guided injections in the musculoskeletal system. *Ultrasound Q* 2003;19(1):3–12.
3. Sofka CM, Adler RS. Ultrasound-guided interventions in the foot and ankle. *Semin Musculoskel Radiol* 2002;6:163–168.
4. Balint PV, Kane D, Hunter J, et al. Ultrasound guided versus conventional joint and soft tissue fluid aspiration in rheumatology practice: a pilot study. *J Rheumatol* 2002; 29:2209–2213.
5. Chiou HJ, Chou YH, Wu JJ, et al. Alternative and effective treatment of shoulder ganglion cyst: ultrasonographically guided aspiration. *J Ultrasound Med* 1999;18:531–535.
6. Breidahl WH, Adler RS. Ultrasound-guided injection of ganglia with corticosteroids. *Skeletal Radiol* 1996;25:635–638.

Subject Index